Biomarkers in Allergy and Asthma

Editors

FLAVIA C.L. HOYTE
ROHIT K. KATIAL

IMMUNOLOGY AND ALLERGY CLINICS OF NORTH AMERICA

www.immunology.theclinics.com

Consulting Editor
STEPHEN A. TILLES

November 2018 • Volume 38 • Number 4

ELSEVIER

1600 John F. Kennedy Boulevard ● Suite 1800 ● Philadelphia, Pennsylvania, 19103-2899

http://www.theclinics.com

IMMUNOLOGY AND ALLERGY CLINICS OF NORTH AMERICA Volume 38, Number 4

November 2018 ISSN 0889-8561, ISBN-13: 978-0-323-64139-5

Editor: Jessica McCool
Developmental Editor: Kristen Helm

Immunology and Allergy Clinics of North America (ISSN 0889–8561) is published quarterly by Elsevier Inc., 360 Park Avenue South, New York, NY 10010-1710. Months of issue are February, May, August, and November. Periodicals postage paid at New York, NY and additional mailing offices. Subscription prices are $333.00 per year for US individuals, $565.00 per year for US institutions, $100.00 per year for US students and residents, $411.00 per year for Canadian individuals, $220.00 per year for Canadian students, $717.00 per year for Canadian institutions, $445.00 per year for international individuals, $717.00 per year for international institutions, $220.00 per year for international students. To receive student/resident rate, orders must be accompanied by name of affiliated institution, date of term, and the *signature* of program/residency coordinator on institution letterhead. Orders will be billed at individual rate until proof of status is received. Foreign air speed delivery is included in all *Clinics* subscription prices. All prices are subject to change without notice. **POSTMASTER:** Send address changes to *Immunology and Allergy Clinics of North America,* Elsevier Health Sciences Division, Subscription Customer Service, 3251 Riverport Lane, Maryland Heights, MO 63043. **Customer Service: 1-800-654-2452 (U.S. and Canada); 314-447-8871 (outside U.S. and Canada). Fax: 314-447-8029. E-mail: journalscustomerservice-usa@elsevier.com (for print support); journalsonlinesupport-usa@elsevier.com (for online support).**

Reprints. For copies of 100 or more, of articles in this publication, please contact the Commercial Reprints Department, Elsevier Inc., 360 Park Avenue South, New York, New York 10010-1710. Tel. 212-633-3874, Fax: 212-633-3820, E-mail: reprints@elsevier.com.

Immunology and Allergy Clinics of North America is covered in MEDLINE/PubMed (Index Medicus), Current Contents/Life Sciences, Science Citation Index, ISI/BIOMED, Chemical Abstracts, and EMBASE/Excerpta Medica.

Contributors

CONSULTING EDITOR

STEPHEN A. TILLES, MD
Executive Director, ASTHMA Inc. Clinical Research Center, Partner, Northwest Asthma and Allergy Center, Clinical Professor of Medicine, University of Washington, Seattle, Washington, USA

EDITORS

FLAVIA C.L. HOYTE, MD
Associate Professor, Director, Fellowship Training Program, Division of Allergy and Immunology, Department of Medicine, National Jewish Health, Denver, Colorado, USA

ROHIT K. KATIAL, MD
Professor, Division of Allergy and Immunology, Department of Medicine, National Jewish Health, Denver, Colorado, USA

AUTHORS

ANURAG BHALLA, MD
Division of Respirology, Firestone Institute for Respiratory Health, St. Joseph's Healthcare, McMaster University, Hamilton, Ontario, Canada

NOAM A. COHEN, MD, PhD
Department of Otorhinolaryngology–Head and Neck Surgery, Division of Rhinology, University of Pennsylvania, Perelman School of Medicine, Philadelphia VA Medical Center, Monell Chemical Senses Center, Philadelphia, Pennsylvania, USA

PASQUALE COMBERIATI, MD
Department of Clinical and Experimental Medicine, Section of Paediatrics, University of Pisa, Italy; Department of Clinical Immunology and Allergology, I.M. Sechenov First Moscow State Medical University, Russia

RONINA A. COVAR, MD
Department of Pediatrics, National Jewish Health, Denver, Colorado, USA

MICHAEL D. DAVIS, RRT, PhD
Assistant Professor, Division of Pulmonary Medicine, Children's Hospital of Richmond at VCU, Richmond, Virginia, USA

CLAIRE EMSON, PhD
MedImmune, Gaithersburg, Maryland, USA

ERWIN W. GELFAND, MD
Division of Cell Biology, Department of Pediatrics, National Jewish Health, Denver, Colorado, USA

LARA M. GROSS, MD
Division of Allergy and Immunology, National Jewish Health, University of Colorado Hospital, Denver, Colorado, USA

BRYCE C. HOFFMAN, MD
Fellow, Department of Pediatrics, Division of Allergy and Immunology, National Jewish Health, Denver, Colorado, USA

FLAVIA C.L. HOYTE, MD
Director, Fellowship Training Program, Division of Allergy and Immunology, Associate Professor, Department of Medicine, National Jewish Health, Denver, Colorado, USA

ROHIT K. KATIAL, MD
Professor, Division of Allergy and Immunology, Department of Medicine, National Jewish Health, Denver, Colorado, USA

MICHAEL A. KOHANSKI, MD, PhD
Department of Otorhinolaryngology–Head and Neck Surgery, Division of Rhinology, University of Pennsylvania, Perelman School of Medicine, Philadelphia, Pennsylvania, USA

SCOTT MANETZ, PhD
MedImmune, Gaithersburg, Maryland, USA

ALISON J. MONTPETIT, RN, PhD
Nurse Clinician – Nurse Scientist, VCU Health Department of Emergency Medicine, Adult Emergency Department, Richmond, Virginia, USA

MANALI MUKHERJEE, PhD
Division of Respirology, Firestone Institute for Respiratory Health, St. Joseph's Healthcare, McMaster University, Hamilton, Ontario, Canada

PARAMESWARAN NAIR, MD, PhD, FRCP, FRCPC
Division of Respirology, Firestone Institute for Respiratory Health, St. Joseph's Healthcare, McMaster University, Hamilton, Ontario, Canada

PAUL NEWBOLD, PhD
MedImmune, Gaithersburg, Maryland, USA

REYNOLD A. PANETTIERI Jr, MD
Professor of Medicine, Robert Wood Johnson Medical School, Vice Chancellor for Translational Medicine and Science, Director, Rutgers Institute for Translational Medicine and Science, Rutgers, The State University of New Jersey, New Brunswick, New Jersey, USA

TUYET-HANG PHAM, MS
MedImmune, Gaithersburg, Maryland, USA

NATHAN RABINOVITCH, MD, MPH
Professor, Department of Pediatrics, Division of Allergy and Immunology, National Jewish Health, Denver, Colorado, USA

NIKITA RAJE, MD
Staff, Allergy/Immunology, Children's Mercy Hospital, University of Missouri-Kansas City School of Medicine, Kansas City, Missouri, USA

NIHARIKA RATH, MD
Fellow, Allergy/Immunology, Children's Mercy Hospital, University of Missouri-Kansas City School of Medicine, Kansas City, Missouri, USA

LANNY ROSENWASSER, MD
Staff, Allergy/Immunology, University of Missouri-Kansas City School of Medicine, Kansas City, Missouri, USA

MICHAELA SCHEDEL, PhD
Division of Cell Biology, Department of Pediatrics, National Jewish Health, Denver, Colorado, USA

ALAN D. WORKMAN, MD, MTR
Department of Otorhinolaryngology–Head and Neck Surgery, Division of Rhinology, University of Pennsylvania, Perelman School of Medicine, Philadelphia, Pennsylvania, USA

Contents

> Bronchial hyperresponsiveness (BHR) is defined as a heightened bronchoconstrictive response to airway stimuli. It complements the cardinal features in asthma, such as variable or reversible airflow limitation and airway inflammation. To what extent the mechanisms of airflow limitation, airway inflammation, and BHR overlap is unclear, and how these 3 components come together probably accounts for the wide variability of asthma. This article covers the relationships between BHR and airway inflammation, describes the latest updates on the use of BHD in the diagnosis and management of asthma, and finally highlights the gaps in our current knowledge relating to BHR in asthma.

> Fractional concentration of exhaled nitric oxide (FENO) is a biomarker used to identify allergic airway inflammation. Because it is noninvasive and easy to obtain, its utility has been studied in the diagnosis and management of several respiratory diseases. Much of the research has been done in asthma, and many studies support the use of FENO in aiding diagnosing asthma, predicting steroid responsiveness, and preventing exacerbations by guiding medication dosage and assessing adherence.

> Asthma is a chronic disease that affects children and adults with significant morbidity and mortality. It is multifactorial, with genetic and environmental factors affecting the overall course of the disease. Both specific and total immunoglobulin (Ig)E can be used in specific phenotypes such as allergic asthma. Using IgE as a biomarker for asthma provides a target for management and treatment. Biotherapeutics continue to emerge as important advances in asthma treatment, and their effect on IgE and its biomarker role continue to be studied.

Measurement of urinary leukotriene E_4 (uLTE_4) is a sensitive and noninvasive method of assaying total body cysteinyl leukotriene (CysLT) production and changes in CysLT production. Recent studies have reported on novel LTE4 receptor interactions and genetic polymorphisms causing CysLT variability. The applications of uLTE_4 as a biomarker continue to expand, including evaluation of environmental exposures, asthma severity risk, aspirin sensitivity, predicting atopy in preschool age children, obstructive sleep apnea, and predicting susceptibility to leukotriene receptor antagonists.

Periostin and dipeptidyl peptidase-4 (DPP-4) are proteins induced by type 2 cytokines interleukin (IL)-4 and IL-13 and show increased expression in asthma and diseases with type 2 inflammation, including atopic dermatitis and chronic rhinosinusitis. Both proteins can also be induced by other stimuli, such as profibrotic factors, which may confound their specificity as biomarkers of IL-13 pathway activation and type 2–driven disease. DPP-4 is important in glucose metabolism; therefore, serum concentrations may be confounded by the presence of concomitant metabolic disease. This review evaluates the potential of these biomarkers for anti–IL-13–directed therapy in asthma and diseases with type 2 inflammation.

Although asthma defines a syndrome associated with airway inflammation, heterogeneity exists concerning the type of inflammation that modulates airway hyperresponsiveness. Compelling evidence suggests that common triggers of asthma exacerbations are preferentially mediated by neutrophilic airway inflammation. Currently, there exists no therapeutic approach that uniquely targets neutrophils in asthma. Given that neutrophilic airway inflammation seems to be steroid insensitive and given recent advances in neutrophil biology, exciting opportunities may lead to targeted therapy that focuses on the activation state of neutrophils rather than neutrophil number as a means to improve asthma outcomes in difficult to treat patients.

Eosinophils are critical in asthma biology, contributing to symptoms, airflow obstruction, airway hyperresponsiveness, and remodeling. In severe asthma, in addition to local maturation in bone marrow, *in situ* eosinophilopoiesis plays a key role in the persistence of airway eosinophilia. Local milieu of structural, epithelial and inflammatory cells contribute by generating eosinophilopoietic cytokines in response to epithelial-derived alarmins. Another mechanism of persistent airway eosinophilia is gluco-corticosteroid insensitivity, which is linked to recurrent airway infections and presence of local autoantibodies. Novel molecules are being developed to target specific immune pathways as potential steroid-sparing strategies.

Diagnosis and management of asthma is commonly implemented based on clinical assessment. Although these nonmolecular biomarkers have been useful, limited resolution of the heterogeneity among asthmatic patients and little information regarding the underlying pathobiology of disease in individuals have been provided. Molecular endotyping using global transcriptome expression profiling associated with clinical features of asthma has improved our understanding of disease mechanisms, risk assessment of asthma exacerbations, and treatment responses, especially in patients with type 2 inflammation. Further advances in establishing pathobiological subgroups, bioactive pathways, and true disease endotypes hold potential for a more personalized medical approach in asthmatic patients.

Exhaled breath condensate (EBC) is a promising source of biomarkers of lung disease. EBC research and utility has increased substantially over the past 2 decades. This review summarizes many of the factors regarding the composition of EBC, its collection, and analysis for the utility of both clinicians and researchers.

Chronic rhinosinusitis is a complex disease that exists along the inflammatory spectrum between types 1 and 2 inflammation. The classic phenotypic differentiation of chronic rhinosinusitis based on the presence or absence of inflammatory polyps remains one of the best differentiators of response to therapy. Development of biologics for the treatment of atopic disease and asthma and topical therapies for sinusitis have placed renewed emphasis on understanding the pathophysiology of polyp disease. Identification of key markers of polyposis will allow for better stratification of inflammatory polyp disease endotypes to objectively identify medical therapies and track response to treatment.

Biomarkers in Allergy and Asthma

IMMUNOLOGY AND ALLERGY CLINICS OF NORTH AMERICA

ISSUE OF RELATED INTEREST

Otolaryngologic Clinics of North America, December 2017 (Vol. 50, No. 6)
Allergy for the Otolaryngologist
Murugappan Ramanathan Jr and James W. Mims, *Editors*
Available at http://www.oto.theclinics.com/

THE CLINICS ARE AVAILABLE ONLINE!
Access your subscription at:
www.theclinics.com

Foreword

Biomarkers in Allergic Diseases and Asthma: Essential Tools for Diagnosis and Treatment

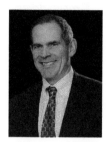

Stephen A. Tilles, MD
Consulting Editor

As our knowledge base has grown, we tend to partition common problems into multiple subcategories based on a "cutting edge" classification system. For example, it was not too many years ago that asthma was classified as either "intrinsic" or "extrinsic." We have come a long way since then, initially dividing diseases into phenotypes based on clinical presentation, and more recently into endotypes based on pathophysiological mechanisms. The evolution of our ability to precisely diagnose diseases has coincided with a growing desire to "personalize" medicine for our patients, and while accurate diagnosis is intellectually satisfying, what really counts is whether our ability to efficiently diagnose diseases can be translated into preventing, curing, or optimally treating those diseases.

Biomarkers are objective measures of biologic processes, and in medicine they have become invaluable both as markers of disease or severity of disease and as a way to direct appropriate therapy. In this issue of the *Immunology and Allergy Clinics of North America*, Drs Hoyte and Katial have assembled a world class group of authors to comprehensively review specific biomarkers used to assess and manage patients with asthma and allergies. I recommend this issue as a "must-have" resource

Immunol Allergy Clin N Am 38 (2018) xi–xii
https://doi.org/10.1016/j.iac.2018.07.002
0889-8561/18/© 2018 Published by Elsevier Inc.

for all practicing allergists and others with an interest in cutting edge approaches to diagnosing and managing allergic diseases.

Stephen A. Tilles, MD
ASTHMA Inc. Clinical Research Center
Northwest Asthma and Allergy Center
University of Washington
9725 3rd Avenue Northeast, Suite 500
Seattle, WA 98115, USA

E-mail address:
stilles@nwasthma.com

Preface

Biomarkers in Allergy and Asthma

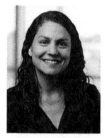 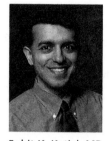

Flavia C.L. Hoyte, MD   Rohit K. Katial, MD
Editors

It is increasingly evident that severe asthma is not a single disease, as evidenced by the variety of clinical presentations, physiologic characteristics, and outcomes seen in patients with asthma. To better understand this heterogeneity, the concept of asthma phenotyping and endotyping has emerged. Phenotyping integrates both biological and clinical features, from molecular, cellular, morphologic, and functional to patient-oriented characteristics with the goal to improve therapy. Ultimately, these phenotypes evolve into asthma "endotypes," which combine clinical characteristics with identifiable mechanistic pathways. Biomarkers, defined as characteristics that can be objectively measured and serve as an indicator of underlying biological processes or pathogenesis, are crucial in defining phenotypes and endotypes.

In asthma, genetic polymorphisms, measures of airway physiology, and levels of inflammatory mediators in urine, blood, sputum, tissue, exhaled gas, and breath condensate have all been studied as potential markers to improve and objectify asthma diagnosis and management. Developing such tools will allow us to phenotype and endotype the various clinical patterns described in asthma, with the ultimate goal of tailoring therapy based on a specific biomarker profile. Biomarkers can then be used to help better understand the pharmacologic response to an intervention and adjust therapy accordingly. This issue, which is an update of our 2012 issue on this topic, provides a comprehensive review of biomarkers that are

Immunol Allergy Clin N Am 38 (2018) xiii–xiv
https://doi.org/10.1016/j.iac.2018.07.001
0889-8561/18/© 2018 Published by Elsevier Inc.

currently available or being studied for future use in the diagnosis and therapy of asthma.

Flavia C.L. Hoyte, MD
Division of Allergy and Clinical Immunology
Department of Medicine
National Jewish Health
1400 Jackson Street
Denver, CO 80206, USA

Rohit K. Katial, MD
Division of Allergy and Clinical Immunology
Department of Medicine
National Jewish Health
1400 Jackson Street
Denver, CO 80206, USA

E-mail addresses:
HoyteF@NJHealth.org (F.C.L. Hoyte)
KatialR@NJHealth.org (R.K. Katial)

Bronchoprovocation Testing in Asthma: An Update

Pasquale Comberiati, MD[a,b], Rohit K. Katial, MD[c],
Ronina A. Covar, MD[c],*

KEYWORDS

- Asthma • Airway inflammation • Airway remodeling
- Bronchoprovocation challenges • Bronchial hyperresponsiveness
- Bronchoprovocation testing

KEY POINTS

- Bronchial hyperresponsiveness (BHR) probably represents several inherent elements of the disease process, such as genetic predisposition, airway inflammation, and airway remodeling.
- Airway inflammation is thought to account for the transient and variable component of BHR, although treatments targeting airway inflammation do not normalize BHR.
- The permanent or persistent component of BHR, particularly to direct stimuli, correlates significantly with structural changes in the airway, such as basement membrane thickness and epithelial damage.
- Treatments significantly eliminating BHR are currently lacking.
- BHR, especially to indirect stimuli, could be a meaningful marker to monitor antiinflammatory treatment efficacy.

INTRODUCTION

Bronchial hyperresponsiveness (BHR) is defined as a heightened bronchoconstrictive response to airway stimuli. It complements the cardinal features in asthma, such as variable or reversible airflow limitation and airway inflammation. To what extent the mechanisms of airflow limitation, airway inflammation, and BHR overlap is still unclear, and how these 3 components come together probably accounts for the wide variability of asthma as a disease.[1,2] Although BHR is considered a pathophysiologic

This article is an update of the previously published article on "Bronchoprovocation Testing in Asthma" in the August 2012 issue of the *Immunology and Allergy Clinics of North America*.
Conflict of Interests: None to declare.
[a] Department of Clinical and Experimental Medicine, Section of Paediatrics, University of Pisa, 56126 Pisa, Italy; [b] Department of Clinical Immunology and Allergology, I.M. Sechenov First Moscow State Medical University, 119991 Moscow, Russia; [c] National Jewish Health, 1400 Jackson Street (J321), Denver, CO 80206, USA
* Corresponding author.
E-mail address: covarr@njhealth.org

hallmark of asthma, it should be acknowledged that this property of the airway is dynamic, because its severity and even presence can vary over time, with disease activity, triggers or specific exposure, and with treatment.[2] In addition, it is important to recognize that there is a component that is not reflective of a specific disease entity. Indeed, BHR has been documented in asymptomatic subjects in the general population and in other diseases, such as chronic obstructive pulmonary diseases, congestive heart failure, cystic fibrosis, bronchitis, allergic rhinitis, and even in healthy subjects.[3–5] Whether its presence in these conditions indicates a common inflammatory process is still poorly understood.

Bronchoprovocation challenges (BPCs), using pharmacologic or physical means to evaluate BHR, have been used to serve a variety of purposes. The most common indication of BPC is when a diagnosis of asthma in either a clinical or a research (clinical trials and epidemiologic) setting is in question (eg, in patients who have suggestive symptoms but no documented airflow limitation). In general, the reliability of the test is more useful in excluding a diagnosis than in confirming one, based on the higher negative predictive value compared with its positive predictive ability.[6,7] This is more relevant in special situations, such as involvement in high-risk occupational tasks and environmental exposure (eg, military, scuba diving); however, because of the overlap in provocation doses causing a reduction in lung function at the time of a challenge between diseased and healthy subjects, setting an absolute level to define a diseased state is difficult.[8]

BPCs are also recommended in the evaluation of a patient suspected of having occupational asthma[9] and exercise-induced respiratory symptoms.[10] Assessment of BHR can also be considered for patients who are suspected of having poor symptom perception or for detecting peculiar physiologic features characteristic of certain asthmatics, such as presence of "excessive" airway closure (characterized by lack of plateau on the dose–response curve).[11] In addition to the utility in complementing the clinical diagnosis of asthma, which has the potential to reduce misdiagnosed or overtreated patients both in primary care settings[12,13] and in patients with severe asthma, BPCs have also become an important research outcome measure to monitor intervention outcome and determine mechanisms underlying efficacy.[1] Finally, there is increasing evidence that BHR can serve as a biomarker to monitor asthma control and adjust antiinflammatory therapy with inhaled corticosteroids (ICSs).[14,15]

BHR is related to various measures of asthma severity,[3,16,17] and it has also been reported as a predictor of development of persistent asthma[18–20] and airflow limitation in adulthood.[21,22] These significant applications of BPCs make them a requirement and in many instances the gold standard in the evaluation of asthma. Hence, it is important to reflect on what these tests convey about asthma.

Central to the application and interpretation of BPCs is the understanding and standardizing of the numerous BPCs available. Recent evidence strongly suggests that various commonly used BPCs differ in their potential to serve as inflammatory biomarkers in relation to whether a direct (eg, methacholine and histamine) or indirect (eg, exercise, adenosine, hypertonic saline, and mannitol) stimulus is used to assess BHR. The response to a direct stimulus depends on the smooth muscle's response to the chemical, whereas in indirect challenges, the reaction is caused by the smooth muscle's responsiveness to the mediators induced by the stimulus. The information obtained from numerous studies with BPCs has provided valuable insights into the pathogenesis and pathophysiology of asthma and the relationships between airway inflammation and BHR.

This article covers the relationships between BHR and airway inflammation and highlights the gaps in our current knowledge relating to BHR in asthma.

WHAT FACTORS CONSTITUTE BRONCHIAL HYPERRESPONSIVENESS?
Genetic Component

Recent "genome-wide association studies" have revealed a substantial number of distinct genetic loci associated with susceptibility to asthma and with several key features of asthma, including lung function, BHR, and disease severity.[23] A genotype-specific difference in response to methacholine was recently noted in a trial assessing response to treatment with salmeterol in combination with ICS, where beta-2 adrenergic receptor genotype seemed to influence improvements in BHR to methacholine following treatment.[24] Furthermore, recent gene expression profiling of airway smooth muscle tissue revealed 8 novel genes that differentiated asthmatic from nonasthmatic patients, 4 of which were related to the severity of BHR.[25]

There is also evidence of genetic susceptibility not only to asthma and atopy, but more specifically to BHR, from clustering of these conditions in families.[26] The narrow-sense heritability of BHR has been reported to be approximately 30%.[27] The association of asthma, atopy, and BHR was stronger between identical twins compared with dizygotic twins. The strong correlation in monozygotic twins suggests an overlap between these genetic factors involved in each of these traits.[28]

Coinheritance and colocalization of a gene to a region of chromosome 5q31–q33 that determines BHR to both histamine and serum immunoglobulin E (IgE) levels have been reported.[29] In that study, elevated levels of serum IgE were coinherited in siblings with BHR, but BHR was not correlated in siblings concordant for elevated serum IgE. These findings suggest that different genetic and environmental factors influence serum IgE levels, not necessarily affecting BHR. There are also several airway inflammatory mediators that are linked to chromosome 5q31–q33, such as granulocyte macrophage colony stimulating factor (GMCSF); fibroblast growth factor-acidic; other colony-stimulating factors and receptors; the lymphocyte-specific glucocorticoid receptor 1; beta-2 adrenergic receptor; and interleukin (IL)-3, IL-4, IL-5, IL-9, and IL-13.[29] Colocalization of these genes in that region may account for the common pathophysiologic features of asthma involving IL-4 in isotype switch to IgE and IL-3, IL-5, and GMCSF for proliferation and activation of eosinophils.

There are other genetic studies that link atopy or serum IgE levels or asthma to BHR, located in other regions such as in chromosome 11[30] and in the IL-4 and IL-13 cytokine region of chromosome 5,[31] more proximal to that found by Postma and colleagues.[29]

These findings still await confirmation in other populations. Currently, the mechanisms linking genetic predisposition and BHR remain to be defined, and no definite gene has been identified to date to account for BHR. In addition, gene–environment interaction may be key in that exposure to early environmental factors (such as passive smoke or other factors related to tobacco smoke in early life, such as viral infections) may modulate the genetic susceptibility for asthma-related phenotype.[32,33]

Transient and Permanent Components of Bronchial Hyperresponsiveness

In asthma, BHR can be variable both within and between individuals. The variability emanates from a different underlying cause in addition to genetic predisposition, which includes presence of airway structural changes that account for more permanent component and the degree or severity of airway inflammation that contributes to the transient or modifiable elements. O'Byrne and Inman[34] proposed the terms persistent and transient, respectively, to differentiate these elements. For example, recent exposures to allergen,[35–38] ozone,[39] infection,[40,41] or occupational triggers[42,43] contribute to the transient property, whereas structural changes affect the permanent or persistent component.

The role of airway smooth muscle in bronchoconstriction and BHR is well recognized, but whether there are unique inherent airway smooth muscle characteristics or whether airway smooth muscle is merely an effector of an abnormal inflammatory response is unclear.[2] Airway inflammation is critical in the pathogenesis of asthma. What specific component of the inflammatory cascade and to what extent inflammation affect BHR are disputed. Furthermore, the physiologic and structural changes characteristic of airway remodeling (ie, fibrosis, smooth muscle hypertrophy, extracellular matrix deposition, vascularity) or epithelial damage[44] probably have a greater impact over airway inflammation on the more permanent feature of BHR.[45] In a double-blind, randomized, placebo-controlled, parallel group study, the relationships between airflow limitation, airway inflammation, airway remodeling, and BHR before and after treatment with high-dose inhaled fluticasone propionate (FP 750 μg twice daily) were evaluated in a group of patients who had mild persistent asthma.[46] Multiple regression analysis indicated that the 40% of the variability in BHR consisted of 21% being related to reticular basement membrane thickness ($P = .009$), 11% to bronchoalveolar lavage epithelial cells ($P = .04$), and 8% to bronchoalveolar lavage eosinophils ($P = .046$), with spirometric indices and mast cells being insignificant predictors of BHR. The longitudinal data validated the cross-sectional model. Spirometric indices and cellular inflammation improved after 3 months of treatment, with no further improvement at 12 months, whereas BHR improved throughout the 1-year study, represented by 6 doubling dose changes. A reduction in reticular basement membrane thickness serving as an index of airway remodeling was evident much later, only after 12 months of treatment (mean change 1.9, 95% confidence interval [CI], 3–0.7 μm; $P = .01$ vs baseline, $P = .05$ vs placebo). Early changes in BHR (ie, 2 doubling dose magnitudes) could be accounted for by improvement in airway inflammation within 3 months and subsequent improvement by airway remodeling.[46] Hence, both airway inflammation and airway remodeling contribute to BHR, and this study provides cross-sectional and longitudinal support that a larger contribution comes from features of airway remodeling. Both features of airway inflammation and remodeling respond, albeit temporally different, to anti-inflammatory treatment with ICS, although BHR did not resolve completely.

Recent findings suggest that ventilation heterogeneity may be another mechanism that contributes to BHR, perhaps from both inflammatory and noninflammatory processes. A causal relationship has been hypothesized by a modeling study, which showed that an uneven distribution of ventilation and airway narrowing throughout the airways resulted in a greater overall increase in airway resistance following uniformly applied bronchoconstriction (ie, BHR).[47] Such results have been strengthened by subsequent studies, which showed that baseline ventilation heterogeneity (measured by the index S_{cond} derived from multiple breath nitrogen washout) is an independent determinant of BHR and strongly correlates with the severity of BHR in patients with asthma.[48,49] Of interest, ventilation heterogeneity seems to be, at least in part, independent of steroid responsive inflammatory process, as a significant correlation with BHR persisted following 3 months of ICS treatment.[48] Whether this residual ventilation heterogeneity is caused by other inflammatory processes, structural changes, or airway remodeling requires further investigation.

What makes the issue more complex is that the actual method of bronchoprovocation testing may provide a diverse relationship between inflammation and BHR. Indirect challenges are presumed to be more reflective of airway inflammation, in contrast to direct stimuli, which are more related to the irreversible or persistent BHR. It is likely that there are many variables contributing to BHR and in specific conditions, different mechanisms or a combination thereof are responsible.

THE LINK BETWEEN BRONCHIAL HYPERRESPONSIVENESS AND AIRWAY INFLAMMATION
Associations Between Bronchial Hyperresponsiveness and Other Inflammatory Biomarkers

Evidence in support of this relationship can be grouped according to associations between inflammatory and allergic markers and BHR, and modification of BHR and inflammatory markers using antiinflammatory medications.

Allergen challenges in animal and human studies using single or repeated doses induce airway reactivity that is associated with a variety of immunologic features, such as production of antigen-specific IgE levels, upregulation of T-helper cytokines, early and late-phase reactions, and eosinophilic inflammation.[50–53] After allergen stimulation, the influx of inflammatory cells in the airways, notably eosinophils, precedes the development of late-phase response and correlates with an increase in BHR. The onslaught of inflammatory cells in the airways at the time of the allergen challenge suggests a causal relationship between BHR and airway inflammation. Whether the effect is caused by activation of eosinophil-releasing substances that can increase reactivity or by the epithelial damage itself, which enhances BHR, is not well established.

Associations between BHR and other inflammatory processes or markers that are not necessarily characteristic of purely eosinophilic process exist. Using an animal model for asthma, mice that had been sensitized with ovalbumin and then challenged repeatedly with ovalbumin aerosols were treated with monoclonal antibodies directed against IL-4, IL-5, interferon gamma (IFNγ), or tumor necrosis factor alpha (TNFα) during the challenge period.[54] The control antibody-treated mice showed hyperresponsiveness to methacholine and presence of eosinophils in bronchoalveolar lavage. Treatment with antibodies to IL-4 or IL-5 did not inhibit BHR, although IL-5 specifically inhibited bronchoalveolar lavage eosinophilia in ovalbumin-challenged mice. In contrast, IFNγ completely abolished, and TNFα partially but not significantly inhibited development of airway hyper-responsiveness in ovalbumin-challenged animals, with neither treatment having an effect on eosinophilia.[54]

In another murine model, the ability to develop BHR also did not correlate with the degree of airway eosinophilia, inflammation, or total serum and ovalbumin-specific IgE levels in genetically different inbred mouse strains (BALB/c, B6D2F1, and C57BL/6).[55] Higher BHR was found in the BALB strain that was associated with lower levels of eosinophils and ovalbumin-specific IgE levels, compared with the B6D2F1 strain. Hence, there is an apparent dissociation between eosinophilia and antigen-specific IgE and BHR. In addition, the genetic background of the mice influenced the development of BHR.

A recent study in adults with allergic asthma evaluating the effects of repeated bronchoconstriction induced by either serial inhaled allergen (dust mite) or methacholine challenges on airway remodeling offered interesting observations. Both inhaled allergen and methacholine challenges promoted airway remodeling in terms of increases in subepithelial collagen band thickness and epithelial mucous glands. Notably, this effect seemed to be dissociated from eosinophilic inflammation, because a similar degree of airway reactivity and remodeling was seen following both challenges, but eosinophils into the airways increased only within the allergen-challenged group.[56]

These observations, specifically that of inhibition of BHR using specific mediators independent of the effect on airway eosinophilia, and the dissociation between airway eosinophilia and BHR, suggest that other mechanisms are involved. T lymphocytes have been shown to play a role in intrinsic, nonatopic BHR and the development of antigen-induced BHR.[57–59] Alveolar macrophages may play a role in the development of nonspecific BHR, because these were the only cell types significantly increased in rats receiving repeated antigen challenges.[60] This is supported by a study in people in whom nonspecific BHR to histamine was closely correlated with elevated eosinophils and macrophages and with the ratio of eosinophils to macrophages.[61] Airway mast cells and eosinophils were found to correlate with BHR in asthmatics treated with corticosteroids.[62] A study by Kelly and colleagues[63] also suggests a relation between bronchial responsiveness and both neutrophil numbers and macrophage activity.

Although still speculative, different immune profiles may be involved in the development of BHR based on atopy. Among nonatopics, elevated allergen-specific and polyclonal IL-10 production, TNFα, and IFNγ were associated with BHR, whereas BHR among atopic individuals was associated with eosinophilia, IL-5, and IgE.[64]

There are numerous epidemiologic and clinical trial studies that present associations, albeit modest, between BHR and features of atopy or other biomarkers of eosinophilic inflammation in the airway (from sputum, bronchoalveolar lavage, and exhaled substances).[61,65–73] The associations with various measures of atopy can be variable. For example, in a study by Jansen and colleagues,[74] eosinophilia (odds ratio [OR] = 2.06, 95% CI, 1.28–3.31) and skin test positivity (OR = 1.66, 95% CI, 1.02–2.71) were both significantly associated with BHR to histamine, but high serum total IgE levels were not (OR = 1.29, 95% CI, 0.81–2.03) associated with BHR in this middle-aged population. In addition, the significant association between BHR and positive skin test pertained to symptomatic subjects only (OR = 5.78, 95% CI, 1.63–20.51), independent of eosinophilia and high serum total IgE levels. In contrast, the relationship between peripheral blood eosinophilia and BHR was the same in asymptomatic subjects and symptomatic subjects.[74] These findings suggest that skin testing, serum total IgE level, and peripheral blood eosinophilia represent different features of the atopic phenotype, with eosinophilia having the most robust association with BHR.

The use of a noninvasive measure of airway inflammation such as exhaled nitric oxide concentrations has been applied clinically in the past decade, especially in children. Exhaled nitric oxide has been correlated with BHR both in corticosteroid naive and treated subjects.[62,75,76] With significant associations reported between exhaled nitric oxide levels and BHR, the feasibility of using exhaled nitric oxide measurements makes it a more attractive surrogate biomarker over BHR; however, the association is still quite modest (with approximately 9%–16% of exhaled nitric oxide variability probably attributable to BHR). Therefore, different mechanisms underlie exhaled nitric oxide measurements and BHR.

Although numerous studies illustrate the link between BHR and various measures of airway inflammation, there are studies that show a lack of an association.[44,77–82] Crimi and colleagues[82] evaluated the relationships between BHR and the number and types of inflammatory cells in the sputum, bronchoalveolar lavage, and bronchial biopsy samples of patients who had mild-to-moderate asthma with sensitization to either house dust mite or animal dander. In this study, no association was found between BHR and the presence of inflammatory cells (eosinophils, neutrophils, lymphocytes, or macrophages) in the airways. It could also be possible that it is not just the presence or number of inflammatory cells per se, but the activation of these cells that would correlate with BHR. Perhaps the correlation between role for eosinophils in allergic inflammation and BHR would be more apparent after an allergen challenge and not necessarily at steady state or baseline.[56,83]

Modifying Bronchial Hyperresponsiveness Using Antiinflammatory, Allergen Avoidance, and Immunomodulatory Therapy

More than just associations of BHR with various markers of airway inflammation, convincing evidence supportive of the premise that BHR is indeed a biomarker of airway inflammation comes from numerous clinical trials demonstrating favorable effects of antiinflammatory medications such as ICSs and leukotriene-modifying agents on BHR and other inflammatory indices.[46,84–87] Despite significantly improving symptoms and decreasing airway inflammation, ICSs produce at best a modest decrease in BHR as measured by histamine or methacholine challenges: a magnitude of 1.5 to 6 doubling dose reduction in BHR.[15,42,86,88,89] This suggests that the effect of treatment on BHR is not absolute, despite normalization of lung function or amelioration of symptoms and inflammation. Leukotriene-modifying agents have been shown to reduce bronchial reactivity.[90–93] A study in preschool children found bronchoprotection (measured by change in airway resistance after cold, dry air challenge) in those treated with montelukast (17%) compared with placebo-treated group (46%). In adolescents and adults, using exercise challenge after 12 weeks of treatment to measure the degree of protection against bronchoconstriction, montelukast therapy was associated with a 47.4% improvement in degree of inhibition using area under the curve, compared with placebo; maximal drop in percentage of forced expiratory volume in 1 s (FEV_1%) was 22% versus 32% in patients on montelukast therapy compared with placebo, respectively. There was no significant difference in doubling dose measurements of methacholine between the 2 groups after 12 weeks of treatment.

Environmental interventions to reduce aeroallergen exposure have also been demonstrated to modify bronchial reactivity.[94,95] Children who lived in a house dust mite–free environment at high altitude for a month was found to have improvement in BPCs using adenosine monophosphate (2.15 doubling dose concentration) and exercise (decrease in FEV_1 of 27% at baseline and 21% after 1 month) but not with direct methacholine challenge.[94]

In contrast to the interventions that target a broader influence on the inflammatory response, specific immunomodulation in human studies has afforded no significant effect on BHR, despite a substantial bearing on inflammatory markers. In a randomized, double-blind, parallel, placebo-controlled study in patients with allergic asthma (ie, sensitized to dust mite, grass pollen, or cat dander),[96] single infusion of anti–IL-5 (either 2.5 mg/kg or 10 mg/kg) failed to modify BHR to histamine before and after allergen challenge 1 week and 1 month after the dose, despite a decrease in peripheral blood and sputum eosinophils. Mepolizumab, a humanized monoclonal antibody against IL-5, has been found to reduce severe exacerbations and improve asthma symptoms and sputum and blood eosinophils in patients with refractory eosinophilic asthma, yet no effects on BHR to methacholine was seen after 1-year treatment.[97] These findings suggest that eosinophilia might not be the prime factor responsible for BHR in allergic asthma, because several inflammatory cells (eg, T cells, mast cells, and eosinophils) contribute to the late asthmatic response. In addition, anti-IgE (omalizumab) treatment for 16 weeks given to adults who have mild-to-moderate asthma afforded a marked reduction in free IgE; IgE positive cells in the airway mucosa; sputum eosinophil count; tissue eosinophils; cells positive for the high-affinity Fc receptor for IgE; CD3+, CD4+, and CD8+ T lymphocytes; B lymphocytes; and cells staining for IL-4, without an effect on BHR to methacholine responsiveness.[98] Similar findings were observed in a subsequent study, which showed that omalizumab reduced the BHR to indirect stimuli (adenosine 5'-monophosphate) after 4 and 12 weeks of treatment, without affecting the response to methacholine.[99] Overall, these studies suggest that, at least in allergic asthma, specific therapy directed at eosinophil or IgE regulation does not obliterate bronchial responsiveness to methacholine.

A proof of concept study targeting mast cell in patients with refractory asthma using KIT inhibition with imatinib demonstrated not only a reduction in mast cell activity (serum and BAL tryptase) but also a significant improvement in BHR using methacholine after 6 months in patients treated with imatinib (1.73 ± 0.60 doubling dose from baseline) compared with placebo (1.07 ± 0.60 doubling dose, $P = .048$).[100]

Antiinflammatory compounds that have broader coverage might be more effective at targeting this outcome. A recent study in adults with mild, stable allergic asthma showed that treatment with the humanized monoclonal immunoglobulin G2λ, AMG 157, which binds with thymic stromal lymphopoietin (TSLP) to inhibit receptor interaction, significantly reduced markers of persisting airway inflammation (ie, the fraction of exhaled nitric oxide; blood and sputum eosinophils) and attenuated not only allergen-induced airway responses, including the early and late asthmatic bronchoconstriction but also BHR to methacholine (1.36 vs 0.66 doubling dose in the AMG 157 vs placebo treated groups, respectively).[101] TSLP is a protein released primarily from epithelial cells in response to irritating stimuli,[102] which is thought to initiate signaling pathways leading to Th2 cell-driven inflammation resulting in the production of proinflammatory cytokines, including IL-5, IL-4, and IL-13. Although the biological mechanisms of AMG 157 have to be unraveled, it is likely that this anti-TSLP treatment acts by exerting a broad inhibition of regulatory networks. These findings suggest that TSLP has a key role not only in bronchoconstrictor responses evoked by the inhalation of allergens but also in maintenance of airway inflammation in patients with allergic asthma. However, at this stage it is unclear whether the reduction in eosinophils counts has a causal association with the inhibition of the allergen-induced responses or whether such changes follow another event responsible for the protective effect. This study also showed the utility of allergen-induced airway responses (including BHR to methacholine) as predictive model for the assessment of efficacy of new potential therapies for asthma.[1]

A summary of potential new treatments for asthma and their effects on BHR is provided in **Table 1**.[103–114] Even if a general association exists between BHR and airway inflammation in asthma, such a relationship is not absolute and is therefore limited, because both measures can be influenced by different factors. It is likely that single measurements of BHR to pharmacologic stimuli cannot provide accurate information on airway inflammation. Depending on the BPC used, they could be suggestive of a different disease or immunologic pathway.

Correlations Between Direct and Indirect Challenges

The manner in which BPCs are conducted can be relevant in defining the association between BHR and airway inflammation; hence the distinction between direct and indirect stimuli is made. BPCs using direct stimuli such as methacholine and histamine provoke bronchoconstriction by acting primarily on airway smooth muscles and also on mucous glands and airway microvasculature. Methacholine (acetyl-b-methylcholine chloride), a synthetic derivative of acetylcholine, binds to specific muscarinic receptors, whereas histamine binds to H1 receptors on the airway smooth muscle. In contrast, indirect challenges use stimuli (eg, physical, osmotic, or pharmacologic) that affect inflammatory and neuronal cells and induce release of mediators or cytokines that cause bronchospasm. Examples of stimuli acting indirectly to assess BHR include exercise, adenosine monophosphate (AMP), dry powder mannitol, and

Table 1
Effect of treatment with potential new treatments for asthma, on allergen-induced early responses, late responses, methacholine airway hyperresponsiveness, and sputum eosinophilia

New Molecule	Dosing	Early Response	Late Response	AHR	Eosinophils
Inhaled heparin disaccharide[103]	Single	No	No	No	No
Inhaled PGE2[104]	Single	Yes	Yes	Yes	Yes
Anti-CD11a[105]	8 wk	No	Yes	No	Yes
Antisense against IL-3, GM-CSF, and CCR3[106]	4 d	Yes	No	No	Yes
CPG-Oligo[107]	4 wk	No	No	No	No
Anti−IL-13[108]	2 wk	Yes	Yes	No	No
PDE4 inhibitor[109]	2 wk	No	Yes	Yes	Yes
Anti−Ox 40L[110]	16 wk	No	No	No	No
α7 nicotinic agonist[111]	9 d	No	No	Yes	No
CysLT1/LT2 antagonist[112]	8 d	Yes	Yes	Yes	Yes
Anti-M1 prime[113]	12 wk	Yes	Yes	No	Yes
Nonsteroid GR agonist[114]	1 wk	No	Yes	Yes	Yes
Anti-TSLP[101]	12 wk	Yes	Yes	Yes	Yes

Abbreviations: AHR, airway hyperresponsiveness; GR, glucocorticoid receptor; No, no statistically significant effect; PGE2, prostaglandin E2; Yes, statistically significant attenuation.

From Nair P, Martin JG, Cockcroft DC, et al. Airway hyperresponsiveness in asthma: measurement and clinical relevance. J Allergy Clin Immunol Pract 2017;5(3):655; with permission.

eucapnic voluntary hyperpnoea (EVH). This section presents correlations between direct and indirect BPC and compares the effects of antiinflammatory therapy in regard to symptoms, markers of airway inflammation, and BHR using direct and indirect airway challenges.

The most common pharmacologic agents used for direct challenges are methacholine and histamine; their pharmacokinetic properties are known, and their safety has long been established. Bronchial responsiveness to methacholine and histamine correlates significantly ($r = 0.9$).[115] BPCs using direct stimuli are considered to be highly sensitive in excluding a diagnosis of current asthma, particularly in patients who have asthma symptoms and normal lung function, but they have a relatively low specificity for asthma. Therefore, positive challenges are consistent with but not entirely diagnostic of asthma and must be interpreted with other features of asthma. A careful decision analysis taking into consideration pretest probability and posttest probability is recommended when interpreting the results, considering the continuous variable using PC_{20} and the overlap in PC_{20} results between healthy and diseased patients (**Fig. 1**).[6]

The pretest probability is an estimate of the likelihood of asthma before the procedure is obtained. The posttest probability is the likelihood of asthma taking into account the pretest probability and the methacholine provocation results, so that the actual PC_{20} results represent the contribution of the BPC to the diagnosis. For example, in an epidemiologic survey of asthma with a randomly selected sample whose medical history is not as detailed, an estimate of prevalence or pretest probability would be 5%. Subjects who would have a PC_{20} of 1 mg/mL could have an approximate 45% posttest likelihood of having asthma. When a patient presents with symptoms, the pretest probability is expectedly higher, so that if the estimate is between 30% and 70%, a PC_{20} of 1 mg/mL could bring the posttest estimate to approximately 90%

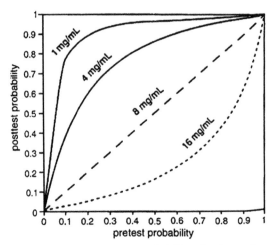

Fig. 1. Curves illustrating pretest and posttest probability of asthma after methacholine challenge test with 4 PC_{20} values. The curves represent a compilation of information from several sources. They are approximations presented to illustrate the relationships and principles of decision analysis. They are not intended to calculate precise posttest probabilities in patients. (*From* Crapo RO, Casaburi R, Coates AL, et al. Guidelines for methacholine and exercise challenge testing - 1999. Am J Respir Crit Care Med 2000;161(1):318; with permission. Copyright © 2000, American Thoracic Society.)

to 98%. The positive predictive value of methacholine challenge for asthma increases the lower PC_{20} (particularly for value <1 mg/mL in the moderate or greater range of BHR) and the higher the pretest probability. False-negative tests should be infrequent if BPC is performed at a time of current or recent symptoms, and potent functional (long-acting beta agonist in particular) or specific (anticholinergic) antagonist medications have been withhold for the appropriate duration prior testing.[116]

The reported sensitivity and specificity of the methacholine challenge test (MCT) has varied depending on the study population tested. In studies with large sample sizes, sensitivity ranged from 51%[117] to 100%[118] and specificity ranged from 49%[119] to 100% (**Table 2**).[117–131] Much of these data are based on older clinical trials. However, the current American Thoracic Society (ATS) guidelines suggest that MCTs can be used to exclude asthma if the PC_{20} is greater than 16 mg/mL in the proper clinical setting.[6] This conclusion was based mainly on studies before ICS use had become a mainstay treatment for asthma. Hence a negative MCT result has been generally interpreted as indicating that it is unlikely that a patient with respiratory symptoms has asthma. A recent study conducted by the Asthma Clinical Research Consortium demonstrated that in 125 asthmatic subjects receiving controller treatment and 92 nonasthmatic control subjects an MCT, sensitivity of 77% and specificity of 96% were observed with a threshold of 8 mg/mL. Increasing the threshold to 16 mg/mL did not substantially increase the sensitivity.[127] In the latter trial, it was also observed that race and the presence of atopy had a significant effect on methacholine sensitivity. The MCT was much less sensitive in white participants (69%) compared with African Americans (91%, $P = .015$).[127]

There are several issues in cross comparing the numerous studies evaluating the performance of the MCT. The study population may differ in several ways, racially, in the severity of asthma, degree of airflow limitation, presence or absence of asthma symptoms, presence of underling atopy and obesity, and use of controller

Table 2
Selected studies evaluating the performance of methacholine challenge tests

Author (Reference), Year	Study Population	No. Adults or Pediatrics	Sensitivity	Specificity	PPV	NPV	Definition of Positive PC$_{20}$ (mg/mL)[a]
Hopp et al,[120] 1984	Asthma, healthy control	165 Pediatrics	98%	63%	57%	99%	800 BU[a]
Cockcroft et al,[118] 1992	College students	500 Adults	100%	93%	34%	100%	8
Nieminen,[123] 1992	Outpatient pulmonary clinic referrals	791 Adults	89%	76%	71%	91%	2600 μg[a]
Perpina et al,[124] 1993	Asthma, rhinitis, chronic bronchitis, healthy control	300 Adults	84%	86%	No information	No information	15
Goldstein et al,[122] 1994	Allergy clinic referrals	198 Adults, pediatrics	61%	100%	100%	74%	8
Goldstein et al,[126] 2001	Suspected asthmatic patients with normal lung function in private clinic	121 Adults, pediatrics	86%	100%	100%	56%	8
Liem et al,[121] 2008	Manitoba birth cohort: asthma, healthy control	640 Pediatrics	66%	64%	No information	No information	4
Anderson et al,[117] 2009	Suspected asthmatic patients recruited from multiple study sites	375 Adults, pediatrics	51%	75%	78%	46%	16
Sverrild et al,[125] 2010	Young adults randomly drawn from nationwide registration in Denmark	238 Adults, pediatrics (age 15–24 y)	69%	80%	49%	90%	8 μmol[a]
Carlsten et al,[119] 2011	Birth cohort with high risk for asthma	348 Pediatrics	80%	49%	27%	92%	3

Abbreviations: BU, breath units; NPV, negative predictive value; PPV, positive predictive value.
[a] These studies used a provocative dose of methacholine to define a positive test result (PD$_{20}$).
From Sumino K, Sugar EA, Irvin CG, et al. Methacholine challenge test: diagnostic characteristics in asthmatic patients receiving controller medications. J Allergy Clin Immunol 2012;130(1):74; with permission.

medications. Finally, it is possible that the method by which the MCT is performed may influence the results. Previous studies and the ATS guidelines on MCTs have indicated that the 2 MCT methods, 5-breath dosimeter and 2-minute tidal breathing, are equivalent.[128–130] However, 2 groups recently reported evidence of a lack of comparability between the 2 methods.[128–132] These investigators found that patients with mild asthma (PC_{20} >2 mg/mL) were more likely to have a positive MCT result with the tidal breathing method than with the 5-breath dosimeter method. The dosimeter method using repeated deep inhalations has been shown to cause bronchoprotective effect and false-negative results, especially in those with milder airway hyperresponsiveness,[133] therefore reducing the diagnostic sensitivity of the test. To allow comparable results from different devices or protocols, the latest European Respiratory Society (ERS) guidelines on methacholine challenge (endorsed by the ATS) recommend to avoid deep-breath methods and to base the test result on the delivered dose of methacholine causing a 20% decrease in FEV_1 (provocative dose [PD_{20}]), rather than using methacholine concentration (PC_{20}).[134] Indeed there is emerging evidence to show that the methacholine dose, expressed as PD_{20}, ideally eliminates the overestimation of dose when evaporation of the output is not considered and allows more consistent correlation than PC_{20} when comparing responses between different protocols.[135,136] Estimated comparison for PC_{20} in mg/mL (when using the English Wright 2-min tidal protocol) and PD_{20} in μg (calculated as described in ERS guidelines) is reported in **Table 3**.[3]

In 2010, the US Food and Drug Administration approved the dry powder mannitol test for determining BHR in patients 6 years of age or older. Mannitol dry powder is delivered in progressively increasing doses (0, 5, 10, 20, 40, 80, 160, 160, 160 mg), with forced expiratory volume in the first second of expiration (FEV_1) measured 1 minute after each dose. A positive response is a 15% reduction in FEV_1 at a total cumulative dose of 635 mg or a 10% reduction in FEV_1 from baseline between doses. The mannitol test has been suggested for confirming a diagnosis of asthma and to follow response to therapy.[137–141] The advantage of the indirect tests over the direct such as methacholine is that they provide information on 2 key features of asthma, airway inflammation and BHR. In addition to a hyper-responsive smooth muscle, a positive response to mannitol or other indirect stimuli indicates both the presence of inflammatory cells and a sufficient concentration of mediators to cause bronchoconstriction. A negative test result indicates a missing element such as insufficient numbers of inflammatory cells or insufficient concentration of mediators or an unresponsive smooth muscle. Examples of negative tests include known asthmatic patients being treated

Table 3
Categorization of airway response to methacholine

PD_{20} μmol (μg)	PC_{20} mgmL^{-1}	Interpretation
>2 (>400)	>16	Normal
0.5–2.0 (100–400)	4–16	Borderline AHR
0.13–0.5 (25–100)	1–4	Mid-AHR
0.03–0.13 (6–25)	0.25–1	Moderate AHR
<0.03 (<6)	<0.25	Marked AHR

Abbreviations: AHR, airway hyperresponsiveness; PC_{20}, provocative concentration causing a 20% fall in FEV_1; PD_{20}, provocative dose causing a 20% fall in FEV_1.

From Coates AL, Wanger J, Cockcroft DW, et al. ERS technical standard on bronchial challenge testing: general considerations and performance of methacholine challenge tests. Eur Respir J 2017;49(5):1601526; with permission.

effectively with ICSs,[142,143] people with eosinophilic bronchitis but no asthma,[144] or people with asymptomatic BHR to methacholine who may have airway injury such as elite athletes.[121,145,146]

Sverrild and colleagues[125] evaluated methacholine and mannitol and reported a specificity of 80.2% (95% CI, 77.1%–82.9%) and 98.4% (95% CI, 96.2%–99.4%), respectively, with a positive predictive value of 48.6% versus 90.4%, whereas the sensitivity was 68.6% (95% CI, 57.1%–78.4%) and 58.8% (95% CI, 50.7%–62.6%), respectively. Other trials have reported a sensitivity range between 50% and 60%, with specificities in the high 90% range. Although the sensitivity does not seem to be very high, it is important to recognize that the benefit of current treatment on BHR, a previous diagnosis, or the period of current asthma has not always been taken into account when reporting the data. For example, the sensitivity of mannitol to identify a physician diagnosis of asthma increased from 59.8% to 89% when those taking inhaled steroids and negative to mannitol were excluded.[147] Overall, the distinct underlying mechanisms between methacholine and mannitol suggest that performing both tests may be useful in charactering different phenotypes of BHR. Indeed, a recent study among community-managed adult asthmatics reported that 14% had BHR only to methacholine, whereas another 16% had responsiveness only to mannitol.[13]

Mannitol challenge seems to be more sensitive for exercise-induced bronchospasm than an exercise challenge but is not as sensitive as desired for diagnosing exercise-induced bronchospasm. However, because of its relatively high specificity, mannitol may serve as a confirmatory test in those with a positive MCT. A comprehensive discussion on this topic is beyond the scope of this article but 2 extensive reviews have been published discussing mannitol challenges.[147,148]

Among asthmatics, in general, an investigation into the relationship between BHR to histamine and exercise illustrated that inhaled direct challenge would be more sensitive than exercise tests at demonstrating increased nonspecific airway reactivity.[149] In that study, 84% of asthmatics had a positive histamine challenge, whereas only half had evidence of a positive exercise test (ie, 10% drop in FEV_1). Despite the high estimate of asthma diagnosis using direct BPCs such as histamine or methacholine in symptomatic patients, this may compare poorly when indirect challenges are used for a specific purpose. For example, a study was undertaken to investigate the relationship between asthma symptoms and BHR to methacholine and EVH, among symptomatic elite summer-sport athletes because of a notable increase in the prevalence of asthma reports among athletes participating in the Olympic games.[150] In that study, athletes who reported asthma symptoms were twice as likely to have a positive response to EVH challenge (50%; mean reduction in FEV_1 −of 25.4% ± 15%), compared with a positive methacholine challenge (18%; mean PD_{20} of 1.69 mmol to 2.05 mmol). Although all subjects with positive methacholine challenge results had positive EVH challenge results, methacholine had a negative predictive value of only 61% and a sensitivity of 36% for identifying those responsive to EVH. These results suggest that EVH is a more sensitive test for the diagnosis of BHR in elite athletes, and the differences in response to the direct and indirect stimuli raise the possibility of a different pathogenesis involved.[150]

Airway cooling associated with vigorous physical exercise has been thought of as a presumptive cause of exercise-induced asthma. The association of airway cooling with airway hyperreactivity is today folded into 2 potential theories: thermal and osmotic hypotheses. Thermal hypothesis refers to cooling of the airways after exercise that is followed by rapid airway warming, which causes vascular congestion, increased permeability, and edema. The osmotic hypothesis implicates evaporated water loss causing hyperosmolality; stimulation of mucosal drying leading to mast cell degranulation; release of inflammatory mediators such as histamine, prostaglandin D2, and the cysteinyl leukotrienes; and ultimately to edema and airway smooth muscle contraction.

Between indirect challenges specifically to hypertonic saline and exercise challenge, the responses to either stimulus seem to track better. From a community-based, cross-sectional survey, 382 children successfully completed a 4.5% hypertonic saline challenge with increasing inhalation periods, and 365 performed a 6-minute standardized, free running exercise challenge. The prevalence of BHR to hypertonic saline was 20.4%. The results showed similar low sensitivity and high specificity values to identify children who had current wheeze, using 4.5% hypertonic saline challenge (47% and 92%, respectively) and a standardized exercise challenge (46% and 88%, respectively). There was a moderate agreement of response to hypertonic saline and to exercise (kappa = 0.43).[151]

There also seem to be differences between direct and indirect stimuli in the evaluation of response to intervention. Patients sensitized to house dust mites, who were transferred to a more favorable environment at high altitude, demonstrated no significant difference in BHR to methacholine challenge but developed a significant improvement in airway response to adenosine monophosphate, indicated by displacement of the dose–response curve to the right by 2 doubling concentrations ($P = .005$) and exercise ($P = .03$).[94] These results demonstrate the discordance in responses to direct and indirect challenges. The improvement in BHR to the indirect stimuli using AMP and exercise in contrast to the lack of response in BHR to methacholine suggests amelioration of airway inflammation following avoidance of house dust aeroallergens.[94]

Indirect challenges compared with direct stimuli may also be more sensitive in detecting changes in airway reactivity with ICS treatment.[84,85,152–155] BHR to methacholine and AMP was compared, as well as induced sputum analysis and exhaled nitric oxide measurements, before and after 2 weeks of treatment with oral or ICSs. Using multiple regression analysis, corticosteroid improvement in AMP PC_{20} correlated negatively with changes in sputum eosinophils, bronchial epithelial cells, and exhaled nitric oxide and positively with changes in sputum lymphocytes. On the other hand, improvement in methacholine PC_{20} correlated negatively with changes in the number of sputum eosinophils and positively with increase in sputum lymphocytes and FEV_1 percentage predicted. There was a stronger correlation between changes in sputum eosinophils and AMP PC_{20} compared with methacholine PC_{20} ($r = -0.43$, $P = .0001$ vs $r = -0.28$, $P = .004$, respectively). The total explained variance of the improvement in BHR was greater for changes in AMP compared with changes for methacholine (36% vs 22%, respectively). These suggest that improvement in BHR to adenosine may better detect changes in airway inflammation than improvement in methacholine PC_{20}. After inhalation of an aqueous solution administered as AMP, it is converted immediately to adenosine by the ubiquitous enzyme 5′-nucleotidase. Adenosine exerts its effects through interaction with specific adenosine (P1) receptors. The exact mechanism of action of AMP on airway wall is not well-defined, but the role of mast cells is crucial based on a variety of inflammatory mediators, such as histamine, prostaglandins, leukotrienes, and IL-8 release, from human mast cells enhanced by adenosine in vitro.[156–159] Although there are studies that have shown differential BHR response to antiinflammatories such as ICSs, there are also those that show concordant effects of these medications on bronchial responsiveness to direct and indirect stimuli.[143,160–163] Perhaps the variability in bronchial response to direct and indirect stimuli from ICS therapy depends not only on the specific drug or stimulant but also on the duration of treatment, dosage, and delivery (see **Table 1**).

Bronchoprovocation Challenges in the Longitudinal Management of Asthma

Current international guidelines on asthma recommend the use of a stepwise management strategy for effective long-term control, with level and adjustment of antiinflammatory pharmacologic treatments based solely on symptoms, lung function, and reliever bronchodilator use.[164–166] Once clinical control is achieved, the dose of ICS should be tapered to the minimal level required to maintain disease control, to minimize side effects associated with their prolonged use. However, this approach may not be adequate, because several studies have shown persisting BHR and airway inflammation in many asthmatics following ICS use despite good clinical control.[46,101,167,168] The presence of ongoing airway inflammation is not only associated with an increased risk of airway remodeling and related long-term loss in lung function[169,170] but it also predicts the risk of future exacerbations and loss of disease control when stepping-down treatment with ICSs.[171,172] In addition, the well-documented flat dose–response curve to ICS for symptoms and lung function with a plateau for improvement above low doses[173] makes these 2 clinical markers insufficient to monitor the effects of antiinflammatory treatments.

Over the past 20 years, there have been many attempts to manage asthma using strategies based on measurements of BHR. In a parallel group study involving 75 adults with mild-to-moderate asthma, Sont and colleagues[174] compared titration of treatment with ICS based either on standard clinical guidelines (symptoms and lung function alone) or additionally on the degree of BHR to methacholine (BHR strategy) over a 2-year period. Participants whose treatment was adjusted based on their BHR had less mild exacerbation (0.23 vs 0.43 exacerbation/year/patient in the control group) and greater improvement in lung function, but required higher doses of ICSs compared with subjects whose treatment was titrated according to recommended clinical guidelines. Of interest, bronchial biopsy findings (available from 49 subjects) showed greater reduction in thickness of the subepithelial reticular layer in the BHR strategy group than in the reference strategy group. The changes in BHR in both strategy groups were correlated with eosinophil counts in the biopsies ($r = -0.48$, $P = .003$). These results provide more indirect but strong evidence of BHR being a surrogate marker of inflammation in asthma. BHR documented as a mean PC_{20} to methacholine of 0.47 mg/mL before treatment was only marginally reduced using the BHR strategy (increase in PC_{20} 1.1 doubling concentrations, not statistically significant).[174] This confirmed previous studies showing that long-term treatment with ICSs does not necessarily normalize BHR to methacholine, emphasizing the limited effects of current pharmacologic therapies on the permanent component of BHR.[170]

A similar study in 206 children (aged 6–16 years) with moderate persistent asthma did not confirm the full clinical benefit of adjusting ICSs dose based on BHR to methacholine. Over a 2-year period, Nuijsink and colleagues[175] found no difference in the number of symptom-free days using the BHR strategy, although a better prebronchodilator FEV_1 was observed in a subgroup of children with allergic asthma. This improvement was also achieved with a higher dose of ICSs in the BHR strategy. This beneficial effect on lung function was lost at follow-up after 3 to 7 years of usual care, when the mean dose of ICSs had diminished from 550 mg/d at the end of the study to 235 mg/d.[176] This suggests that a BHR-guided treatment strategy may need to be sustained in order to preserve lung function. Moreover, as with the study by Sont and colleagues, BHR persisted at the end of the study and did not differ between the treatment groups.

Koenig and colleagues[177] found similar results in adults with mild-to-moderate asthma, although over a shorter duration of treatment (40 weeks), with suboptimal retention rate (70%). BHR strategy with dose adjustment every 8 weeks (instead of every 12 weeks as the Sont and colleagues[174] study) led to use of higher doses of ICSs (either with or without the combination of a long-acting B2-agonist) with no difference in symptom-free days, lung function, albuterol use, and airway responsiveness compared with reference strategy groups.

BHR to indirect stimuli correlates better with airway inflammation and may represent a more clinically relevant marker to guide adjustment of antiinflammatory treatment and monitor asthma control. It is well documented that the regular use of ICSs attenuates or even abolish the airway reactivity to indirect stimuli.[143,178] On the other hand, increase in BHR to mannitol and AMP after stepping down of ICSs in clinically controlled asthmatics has been shown to predict the risk of a subsequent exacerbation and failure of dose reduction.[142,179] Moreover, BHR to mannitol has shown advantages over other current biomarkers of airway inflammation, because it can also be present in asthmatics with noneosinophilic inflammatory phenotypes and normal FeNO level.[180] Given these observations, a recent randomized controlled trial investigated whether tracking BHR to mannitol (using the lower PD10 threshold) could perform better in the management of adults with mild-to-moderate asthma in primary care setting receiving inhaled ciclesonide, compared with twice monthly clinical or spirometric assessments (standard care).[181] Over a period of 12 months, patients managed on the basis of mannitol BHR experienced fewer mild (but not severe) exacerbations and significant improvement not only in symptoms and reliever bronchodilator use but also in BHR to mannitol and methacholine and airway inflammation measured by FeNO levels. However, in keeping with previous findings, the BHR strategy resulted in exposure to a two-fold higher dose of ciclesonide, albeit no significant adrenal suppression (measured by urinary cortisol) was seen compared with the lower doses in the reference strategy group.[181]

Overall, higher ICS doses are needed to affect BHR than that required to achieve clinical improvement. This was recently confirmed in post hoc pooled analysis of data from 4 randomized clinical trials, which demonstrated a dose-response for improvement in both inflammatory outcomes (ie, FeNO, serum eosinophilic cationic protein, and blood eosinophil) and BHR, when using ICSs above low doses (up to 800 mg/d, beclomethasone equivalent), but not for symptoms and lung function.[173] Further prospective studies are warranted to define whether asthma can be controlled better, safely, and more economically using treatment strategies aimed at reducing BHR.

SUMMARY

BHR is an important feature of asthma, and it is considered a useful tool in the diagnosis, monitoring, managing, and prognostication of a complex condition. With its many valuable uses, it probably represents several inherent elements of the disease process, such as genetic predisposition, airway inflammation, structural changes, and airway remodeling. Airway inflammation seems to account for the transient and variable component of BHR. Associations between BHR to direct and indirect stimuli and inflammatory markers are present. In addition, antiinflammatory treatment can reduce airway inflammation and BHR but not close to eliminating it completely. The exact mechanisms that explain the association between BHR and airway inflammation are unknown. The permanent or persistent component of BHR, particularly to direct stimuli, correlates significantly with structural changes in the airway, such as basement membrane thickness and epithelial damage. It might be this component that is resistant or refractory to the effects of available interventions. A few trials of specific immunomodulatory therapy have shown considerable improvements in markers of airway inflammation, without significantly modifying airway reactivity. On the other hand, the inflammatory component may explain the variable component that modulates over time and with antiinflammatory therapy and thus is better reflected by the BHR measured with indirect challenges such as mannitol or exercise or EVH. There is certainly a need to develop interventions that will affect the more permanent feature of BHR. There is also a need to include biomarker measurements in the routine management and surveillance of asthma to improve long-term control. BHR, particularly to indirect stimuli, may provide a reliable marker to best manage asthma in addition to currently recommended clinical monitoring, although further prospective studies are needed to clearly define its role.

REFERENCES

1. Nair P, Martin JG, Cockcroft DC, et al. Airway hyperresponsiveness in asthma: measurement and clinical relevance. J Allergy Clin Immunol Pract 2017;5(3): 649–59.
2. Chapman DG, Irvin CG. Mechanisms of airway hyper-responsiveness in asthma: the past, present and yet to come. Clin Exp Allergy 2015;45(4):706–19.
3. Woolcock AJ, Peat JK, Salome CM, et al. Prevalence of bronchial hyperresponsiveness and asthma in a rural adult population. Thorax 1987;42(5):361–8.
4. Peat JK, Toelle BG, Marks GB, et al. Continuing the debate about measuring asthma in population studies. Thorax 2001;56:406–11.
5. Hospers JJ, Postma DS, Rijcken B, et al. Histamine airway hyper-responsiveness and mortality from chronic obstructive pulmonary disease: a cohort study. Lancet 2000;356:1313–7.
6. Crapo RO, Casaburi R, Coates AL, et al. Guidelines for methacholine and exercise challenge testing-1999. This official statement of the American Thoracic Society was adopted by the ATS Board of Directors, July 1999. Am J Respir Crit Care Med 2000;161(1):309–29.
7. Rijcken B, Schouten JP, Weiss ST, et al. Long term variability of bronchial responsiveness to histamine in a random population sample of adults. Am Rev Respir Dis 1993;148:944–94.
8. Cockcroft DW, Berscheid BA, Murdock KY. Unimodal distribution of bronchial responsiveness to inhaled histamine in a random human population. Chest 1983;83(5):751–4.
9. Vandenplas O, Suojalehto H, Aasen TB, et al. Specific inhalation challenge in the diagnosis of occupational asthma: consensus statement. Eur Respir J 2014;43(6):1573–87.
10. Weiler JM, Brannan JD, Randolph CC, et al. Exercise-induced bronchoconstriction update-2016. J Allergy Clin Immunol 2016;138(5):1292–5.
11. Busse WW, Wanner A, Adams K, et al. Investigative bronchoprovocation and bronchoscopy in airway diseases. Am J Respir Crit Care Med 2005;172(7):807–16.
12. Aaron SD, Vandemheen KL, FitzGerald JM, et al. Reevaluation of diagnosis in adults with physician-diagnosed asthma. JAMA 2017;317(3):269–79.
13. Manoharan A, Lipworth BJ, Craig E, et al. The potential role of direct and indirect bronchial challenge testing to identify overtreatment of community managed asthma. Clin Exp Allergy 2014;44(10):1240–5.

14. Galera R, Casitas R, Martínez-Cerón E, et al. Does airway hyperresponsiveness monitoring lead to improved asthma control? Clin Exp Allergy 2015;45(9): 1396–405.
15. Brannan JD. Bronchial hyperresponsiveness in the assessment of asthma control: Airway hyperresponsiveness in asthma: its measurement and clinical significance. Chest 2010;138(2 Suppl):11S–7S.
16. Josephs LK, Gregg I, Mullee MA, et al. Nonspecific bronchial reactivity and its relationship to the clinical expression of asthma. A longitudinal study. Am Rev Respir Dis 1989;140:350–7.
17. Weiss ST, Van Natta ML, Zeiger RS. Relationship between increased airway responsiveness and asthma severity in the childhood asthma management program. Am J Respir Crit Care Med 2000;162:50–6.
18. Westerhof GA, Coumou H, de Nijs SB, et al. Clinical predictors of remission and persistence of adult-onset asthma. J Allergy Clin Immunol 2018 Jan;141(1): 104–9.
19. Sears MR, Greene JM, Willan AR, et al. A longitudinal, population based, cohort study of childhood asthma followed to adulthood. N Engl J Med 2003;349:1414–22.
20. Jansen DF, Schouten JP, Vonk JM, et al. Smoking and airway hyperresponsiveness especially in the presence of blood eosinophilia increase the risk to develop respiratory symptoms: a 25-year follow-up study in the general adult population. Am J Respir Crit Care Med 1999;160:259–64.
21. Brutsche MH, Downs SH, Schindler C, et al. Bronchial hyperresponsiveness and the development of asthma and COPD in asymptomatic individuals: SAPALDIA cohort study. Thorax 2006;61:671–7.
22. Rasmussen F, Taylor DR, Flannery EM, et al. Risk factors for airway remodeling in asthma manifested by a low postbronchodilator FEV1/vital capacity ratio: a longitudinal population study from childhood to adulthood. Am J Respir Crit Care Med 2002;165(11):1480–8.
23. Portelli MA, Hodge E, Sayers I. Genetic risk factors for the development of allergic disease identified by genome-wide association. Clin Exp Allergy 2015;45:21–31.
24. Wechsler ME, Kunselman SJ, Chinchilli VM, et al. Effect of beta2-adrenergic receptor polymorphism on response to longacting beta2 agonist in asthma (LARGE trial): a genotype stratified, randomised, placebo-controlled, crossover trial. Lancet 2009;374:1754–64.
25. Yick CY, Zwinderman AH, Kunst PW, et al. Gene expression profiling of laser microdissected airway smooth muscle tissue in asthma and atopy. Allergy 2014; 69:1233–40.
26. Hopp RJ, Bewtra AK, Biven R, et al. Bronchial reactivity pattern in nonasthmatic parents of asthmatics. Ann Allergy 1988;61(3):184–6.
27. Palmer LJ, Burton PR, James AL, et al. Familial aggregation and heritability of asthma-associated quantitative traits in a population-based sample of nuclear families. Eur J Hum Genet 2000;8:853–60.
28. Clarke JR, Jenkins MA, Hopper JL, et al. Evidence for genetic associations between asthma, atopy, and bronchial hyperresponsiveness: a study of 8- to 18-yr-old twins. Am J Respir Crit Care Med 2000;162(6):2188–93.
29. Postma DS, Bleecker ER, Amelung PJ, et al. Genetic susceptibility to asthmad-bronchial hyperresponsiveness coinherited with a major gene for atopy. N Engl J Med 1995;333(14):894–900.
30. Ruffilli A, Bonini S. Susceptibility genes for allergy and asthma. Allergy 1997; 52(3):256–73.

31. Marsh DG, Neely JD, Breazeale DR, et al. Linkage analysis of IL4 and other chromosome 5q31.1 markers and total serum immunoglobulin E concentration. Science 1994;264(5162):1152–6.
32. Meyers DA, Postma DS, Stine OC, et al. Genome screen for asthma and bronchial hyper-responsiveness: interactions with passive smoke exposure. J Allergy Clin Immunol 2005;115(6):1169–75.
33. Colilla S, Nicolae D, Pluzhnikov A, et al, Collaborative Study for the Genetics of Asthma. Evidence for gene–environment interactions in a linkage study of asthma and smoking exposure. J Allergy Clin Immunol 2003;111(4):840–6.
34. O'byrne PM, Inman MD. Airway hyperresponsiveness. Chest 2003;123:411S–6S.
35. Cartier A, Thomson NC, Frith PA, et al. Allergen-induced increase in bronchial responsiveness to histamine: relationship to the late asthmatic response and change in airway caliber. J Allergy Clin Immunol 1982;70(3):170–7.
36. De Monchy JG, Kauman HF, Venge P, et al. Bronchoalveolar eosinophilia during allergen-induced late asthmatic reactions. Am Rev Respir Dis 1985;131(3):373–6.
37. Pin I, Freitag AP, O'Byrne PM, et al. Changes in the cellular profile of induced sputum after allergen-induced asthmatic responses. Am Rev Respir Dis 1992;145(6):1265–9.
38. Metzger WJ, Richerson HB, Worden K, et al. Bronchoalveolar lavage of allergic asthmatic patients following allergen bronchoprovocation. Chest 1986;89(4):477–83.
39. O'Byrne PM, Walters EH, Gold BD, et al. Neutrophil depletion inhibits airway hyperresponsiveness induced by ozone exposure. Am Rev Respir Dis 1984;130(2):214–9.
40. Empey DW, Laitinen LA, Jacobs L, et al. Mechanisms of bronchial hyperreactivity in normal subjects after upper respiratory tract infection. Am Rev Respir Dis 1976;113(2):131–9.
41. Laitinen LA, Elkin RB, Empey DW, et al. Bronchial hyperresponsiveness in normal subjects during attenuated influenza virus infection. Am Rev Respir Dis 1991;143(2):358–61.
42. Mapp C, Boschetto P, dal Vecchio L, et al. Protective effect of antiasthma drugs on late asthmatic reactions and increased airway responsiveness induced by toluene diisocyanate in sensitized subjects. Am Rev Respir Dis 1987;136(6):1403–7.
43. Fabbri LM, Boschetto P, Zocca E, et al. Bronchoalveolar neutrophilia during late asthmatic reactions induced by toluene diisocyanate. Am Rev Respir Dis 1987;136(1):36–42.
44. Jeffery PK, Wardlaw AJ, Nelson FC, et al. Bronchial biopsies in asthma. An ultrastructural, quantitative study and correlation with hyperreactivity. Am Rev Respir Dis 1989;140(6):1745–53.
45. Boulet LP, Laviolette M, Turcotte H, et al. Bronchial subepithelial fibrosis correlates with airway responsiveness to methacholine. Chest 1997;112(1):45–52.
46. Ward C, Pais M, Bish R, et al. Airway inflammation, basement membrane thickening and bronchial hyperresponsiveness in asthma. Thorax 2002;57(4):309–16. XA.
47. Venegas JG, Winkler T, Musch G, et al. Self-organized patchiness in asthma as a prelude to catastrophic shifts. Nature 2005;434:777–82.
48. Downie SR, Salome CM, Verbanck S, et al. Ventilation heterogeneity is a major determinant of airway hyperresponsiveness in asthma, independent of airway inflammation. Thorax 2007;62:684–9.

49. Kaminsky DA, Daud A, Chapman DG. Relationship between the baseline alveolar volume-to-total lung capacity ratio and airway responsiveness. Respirology 2014;19:1046–51.

50. Elwood W, Barnes PJ, Chung KF. Airway hyperresponsiveness is associated with inflammatory cell infiltration in allergic brown Norway rats. Int Arch Allergy Immunol 1992;99(1):91–7.

51. Elwood W, Lötvall JO, Barnes PJ, et al. Characterization of allergen-induced bronchial hyperresponsiveness and airway inflammation in actively sensitized brown-Norway rats. J Allergy Clin Immunol 1991;88(6):951–60.

52. Boulet LP, Cartier A, Thomson NC, et al. Asthma and increases in nonallergic bronchial responsiveness from seasonal pollen exposure. J Allergy Clin Immunol 1983;71(4):399–406.

53. Palmqvist M, Pettersson K, Sjostrand M, et al. Mild experimental exacerbation of asthma induced by individualised low-dose repeated allergen exposure. A double-blind evaluation. Respir Med 1998;92(10):1223–30.

54. Hessel EM, Van Oosterhout AJ, Van Ark I, et al. Development of airway hyperresponsiveness is dependent on interferon–γ amma and independent of eosinophil infiltration. Am J Respir Cell Mol Biol 1997;16(3):325–34.

55. Wilder JA, Collie DD, Wilson BS, et al. Dissociation of airway hyperresponsiveness from immunoglobulin E and airway eosinophilia in a murine model of allergic asthma. Am J Respir Cell Mol Biol 1999;20(6):1326–34.

56. Grainge CL, Lau LC, Ward JA, et al. Effect of bronchoconstriction on airway remodeling in asthma. N Engl J Med 2011;364(21):2006–15.

57. De Sanctis GT, Itoh A, Green FH, et al. T-lymphocytes regulate genetically determined airway hyperresponsiveness in mice. Nat Med 1997;3(4):460–2.

58. Gavett SH, Chen X, Finkelman F, et al. Depletion of murine CD4þT lymphocytes prevents antigen-induced airway hyperreactivity and pulmonary eosinophilia. Am J Respir Cell Mol Biol 1994;10(6):587–93.

59. Krinzman SJ, De Sanctis GT, Cernadas M, et al. Inhibition of T cell costimulation abrogates airway hyperresponsiveness in a murine model. J Clin Invest 1996; 98(12):2693–9.

60. Kamachi A, Nasuhara Y, Nishimura M, et al. Dissociation between airway responsiveness to methacholine and responsiveness to antigen. Eur Respir J 2002;19(1):76–83.

61. Ferguson AC, Wong FW. Bronchial hyperresponsiveness in asthmatic children. Correlation with macrophages and eosinophils in broncholavage fluid. Chest 1989;96:988–91.

62. Gibson PG, Saltos N, Borgas T. Airway mast cells and eosinophils correlate with clinical severity and airway hyperresponsiveness in corticosteroid-treated asthma. J Allergy Clin Immunol 2000;105(4):752–9.

63. Kelly C, Ward C, Stenton CS, et al. Number and activity of inflammatory cells in bronchoalveolar lavage fluid in asthma and their relation to airway responsiveness. Thorax 1988;43:684–92.

64. Heaton T, Rowe J, Turner S, et al. An immunoepidemiological approach to asthma: identification of in-vitro T-cell response patterns associated with different wheezing phenotypes in children. Lancet 2005;365(9454):142–9.

65. Kirby JG, Hargreave FE, Gleich GJ, et al. Bronchoalveolar cell profiles of asthmatic and nonasthmatic subjects. Am Rev Respir Dis 1987;136(2):379–83.

66. Wardlaw AJ, Dunnette S, Gleich GJ, et al. Eosinophils and mast cells in bronchoalveolar lavage in subjects with mild asthma. Relationship to bronchial hyperreactivity. Am Rev Respir Dis 1988;137(1):62–9.

67. Pliss LB, Ingenito EP, Ingram RH Jr. Responsiveness, inflammation, and effects of deep breaths on obstruction in mild asthma. J Appl Physiol (1985) 1989; 66(5):2298–304.
68. Woolley KL, Adelroth E, Woolley MJ, et al. Granulocyte-macrophage colony-stimulating factor, eosinophils and eosinophil cationic protein in subjects with and without mild, stable, atopic asthma. Eur Respir J 1994;7(9):1576–84.
69. Bradley BL, Azzawi M, Jacobson M, et al. Eosinophils, T-lymphocytes, mast cells, neutrophils, and macrophages in bronchial biopsy specimens from atopic subjects with asthma: comparison with biopsy specimens from atopic subjects without asthma and normal control subjects and relationship to bronchial hyper-responsiveness. J Allergy Clin Immunol 1991;88(4):661–74.
70. Chetta A, Foresi A, Del Donno M, et al. Bronchial responsiveness to distilled water and methacholine and its relationship to inflammation and remodeling of the airways in asthma. Am J Respir Crit Care Med 1996;153:910–7.
71. Pin I, Radford S, Kolendowicz R, et al. Airway inflammation in symptomatic and asymptomatic children with methacholine hyperresponsiveness. Eur Respir J 1993;6(9):1249–56.
72. Pizzichini E, Pizzichini MM, Efthimiadis A, et al. Indices of airway inflammation in induced sputum: reproducibility and validity of cell and fluid-phase measurements. Am J Respir Crit Care Med 1996;154(2 Pt 1):308–17.
73. Foresi A, Leone C, Pelucchi A, et al. Eosinophils, mast cells, and basophils in induced sputum from patients with seasonal allergic rhinitis and perennial asthma: relationship to methacholine responsiveness. J Allergy Clin Immunol 1997;100(1):58–64.
74. Jansen DF, Rijcken B, Schouten JP, et al. The relationship of skin test positivity, high serum total IgE levels, and peripheral blood eosinophilia to symptomatic and asymptomatic airway hyperresponsiveness. Am J Respir Crit Care Med 1999;159(3):924–31.
75. Jatakanon A, Lim S, Kharitonov SA, et al. Correlation between exhaled nitric oxide, sputum eosinophils, and methacholine responsiveness in patients with mild asthma. Thorax 1998;53(2):91–5.
76. Reid DW, Johns DP, Feltis B, et al. Exhaled nitric oxide continues to reflect airway hyper-responsiveness and disease activity in inhaled corticosteroid-treated adult asthmatic patients. Respirology 2003;8(4):479–86.
77. Chan-Yeung M, Leriche J, Maclean L, et al. Comparison of cellular and protein changes in bronchial lavage fluid of symptomatic and asymptomatic patients with red cedar asthma on follow-up examination. Clin Allergy 1988; 18(4):359–65.
78. Djukanović R, Wilson JW, Britten KM, et al. Quantitation of mast cells and eosinophils in the bronchial mucosa of symptomatic atopic asthmatics and healthy control subjects using immunohistochemistry. Am Rev Respir Dis 1990;142(4): 863–71.
79. Adelroth E, Rosenhall L, Johansson SA, et al. Inflammatory cells and eosinophilic activity in asthmatics investigated by bronchoalveolar lavage. The effects of antiasthmatic treatment with budesonide or terbutaline. Am Rev Respir Dis 1990;142(1):91–9.
80. Ollerenshaw SL, Woolcock AJ. Characteristics of the inflammation in biopsies from large airways of subjects with asthma and subjects with chronic airflow limitation. Am Rev Respir Dis 1992;145(4 Pt 1):922–7.
81. Iredale MJ, Wanklyn SA, Phillips IP, et al. Non-invasive assessment of bronchial inflammation in asthma: no correlation between eosinophilia of induced sputum

and bronchial responsiveness to inhaled hypertonic saline. Clin Exp Allergy 1994;24(10):940–5.

82. Crimi E, Spanevello A, Neri M, et al. Dissociation between airway inflammation and airway hyperresponsiveness in allergic asthma. Am J Respir Crit Care Med 1998;157(1):4–9.

83. Oddera S, Silvestri M, Penna R, et al. Airway eosinophilic inflammation and bronchial hyperresponsiveness after allergen inhalation challenge in asthma. Lung 1998;176(4):237–47.

84. Meijer RJ, Kerstjens HA, Arends LR, et al. Effects of inhaled fluticasone and oral prednisolone on clinical and inflammatory parameters in patients with asthma. Thorax 1999;54(10):894–9.

85. Nielsen KG, Bisgaard H. The effect of inhaled budesonide on symptoms, lung function, and cold air and methacholine responsiveness in 2-to 5-year-old asthmatic children. Am J Respir Crit Care Med 2000;162(4 Pt 1):1500–6.

86. van den Berge M, Kerstjens HA, Meijer RJ, et al. Corticosteroid-induced improvement in the PC20 of adenosine monophosphate is more closely associated with reduction in airway inflammation than improvement in the PC20 of methacholine. Am J Respir Crit Care Med 2001;164(7):1127–32.

87. The Childhood Asthma Management Program Research Group. Long-term effects of budesonide or nedocromil in children with asthma. N Engl J Med 2000;343(15):1054–63.

88. Juniper EF, Kline PA, Vanzieleghem MA, et al. Effect of long-term treatment with an inhaled corticosteroid (budesonide) on airway hyperresponsiveness and clinical asthma in nonsteroid-dependent asthmatics. Am Rev Respir Dis 1990; 142:832–6.

89. Kerrebijn KF, van Essen-Zandvliet EE, Neijens HJ. Effect of long-term treatment with inhaled corticosteroids and beta-agonists on the bronchial responsiveness in children with asthma. J Allergy Clin Immunol 1987;79:653–9.

90. Bisgaard H, Nielsen KG. Bronchoprotection with a leukotriene receptor antagonist in asthmatic preschool children. Am J Respir Crit Care Med 2000;162(1): 187–90.

91. Le JA, Busse WW, Pearlman D, et al. Montelukast, a leukotriene-receptor antagonist, for the treatment of mild asthma and exercise-induced bronchoconstriction. N Engl J Med 1998;339(3):147–52.

92. Kononowa N, Michel S, Miedinger D, et al. Effects of add-on montelukast on airway hyperresponsiveness in patients with well controlled asthma: a pilot study. J Drug Assess 2013;2:49–57.

93. Fischer AR, McFadden CA, Frantz R, et al. Effect of chronic 5-lipoxygenase inhibition on airway hyperresponsiveness in asthmatic subjects. Am J Respir Crit Care Med 1995;152:1203–7.

94. Benckhuijsen J, van den Bos JW, van Velzen E, et al. Differences in the effect of allergen avoidance on bronchial hyperresponsiveness as measured by methacholine, adenosine 5'monophosphate, and exercise in asthmatic children. Pediatr Pulmonol 1996;22(3):147–53.

95. van Velzen E, van den Bos JW, Benckhuijsen JA, et al. Effect of allergen avoidance at high altitude on direct and indirect bronchial hyperresponsiveness and markers of inflammation in children with allergic asthma. Thorax 1996;51(6): 582–4.

96. Leckie MJ, ten Brinke A, Khan J, et al. Effects of an interleukin-5 blocking monoclonal antibody on eosinophils, airway hyperresponsiveness, and the late asthmatic response. Lancet 2000;356(9248):2144–8.

97. Haldar P, Brightling CE, Hargadon B, et al. Mepolizumab and exacerbations of refractory eosinophilic asthma. N Engl J Med 2009;360(10):973.

98. Djukanović R, Wilson SJ, Kraft M, et al. Effects of treatment with anti-immunoglobulin E antibody omalizumab on airway inflammation in allergic asthma. Am J Respir Crit Care Med 2004;170(6):583–93.

99. Prieto L, Gutiérrez V, Colás C, et al. Effect of omalizumab on adenosine 5'-monophosphate responsiveness in subjects with allergic asthma. Int Arch Allergy Immunol 2006;139(2):122–31.

100. Cahill KN, Katz HR, Cui J, et al. KIT inhibition by imatinib in patients with severe refractory asthma. N Engl J Med 2017;376(20):1911–20.

101. Gauvreau GM, O'Byrne PM, Boulet L-P, et al. Effects of an anti-TSLP antibody on allergen-induced asthmatic responses. N Engl J Med 2014;370:2102–10.

102. Allakhverdi Z, Comeau MR, Jessup HK, et al. Thymic stromal lymphopoietin is released by human epithelial cells in response to microbes, trauma, or inflammation and potently activates mast cells. J Exp Med 2007;204:253–8.

103. Duong M, Cockcroft D, Boulet LP, et al. The effect of IVX-0142, a heparin-derived hypersulfated disaccharide, on the allergic airway responses in asthma. Allergy 2008;63:1195–201.

104. Gauvreau GM, Watson RM, O'Byrne PM. Protective effects of inhaled PGE2 on allergen-induced airway responses and airway inflammation. Am J Respir Crit Care Med 1999;159:31–6.

105. Gauvreau GM, Becker AB, Boulet LP, et al. The effects of an anti-CD11a mAb, efalizumab, on allergen-induced airway responses and airway inflammation in subjects with atopic asthma. J Allergy Clin Immunol 2003;112:331–8.

106. Gauvreau GM, Boulet LP, Cockcroft DW, et al. Antisense therapy against CCR3 and the common beta chain attenuates allergen-induced eosinophilic responses. Am J Respir Crit Care Med 2008;177:952–8.

107. Gauvreau GM, Hessel EM, Boulet LP, et al. Immunostimulatory sequences regulate interferon-inducible genes but not allergic airway responses. Am J Respir Crit Care Med 2006;174:15–20.

108. Gauvreau GM, Boulet LP, Cockcroft DW, et al. Effects of interleukin-13 blockade on allergen-induced airway responses in mild atopic asthma. Am J Respir Crit Care Med 2011;183:1007–14.

109. Gauvreau GM, Boulet LP, Schmid-Wirlitsch C, et al. Roflumilast attenuates allergen-induced inflammation in mild asthmatic subjects. Respir Res 2011; 12:140.

110. Gauvreau GM, Boulet LP, Cockcroft DW, et al. OX40L blockade and allergen-induced airway responses in subjects with mild asthma. Clin Exp Allergy 2014;44:29–37.

111. Boulet LP, Gauvreau GM, Cockcroft DW, et al. Effects of ASM-024, a modulator of acetylcholine receptor function, on airway responsiveness and allergen-induced responses in patients with mild asthma. Can Respir J 2015;22:230–4.

112. Gauvreau GM, Boulet LP, FitzGerald JM, et al. A dual CysLT1/2 antagonist attenuates allergen-induced airway responses in subjects with mild allergic asthma. Allergy 2016;71:1721–7.

113. Gauvreau GM, Harris JM, Boulet LP, et al. Targeting membrane-expressed IgE B cell receptor with an antibody to the M1 prime epitope reduces IgE production. Sci Transl Med 6, 243ra85. Ann Neurosci 2014;21(4):150.

114. Gauvreau GM, Boulet LP, Leigh R, et al. A nonsteroidal glucocorticoid receptor agonist inhibits allergen-induced late asthmatic responses. Am J Respir Crit Care Med 2015;191:161–7.

115. Juniper EF, Frith PA, Dunnett C, et al. Reproducibility and comparison of responses to inhaled histamine and methacholine. Thorax 1978;33:705–10.
116. Cockcroft DW. Direct challenge tests. Chest 2010;138:18S–24S.
117. Anderson SD, Charlton B, Weiler JM, et al. Comparison of mannitol and methacholine to predict exercise-induced bronchoconstriction and a clinical diagnosis of asthma. Respir Res 2009;10:4.
118. Cockcroft DW, Murdock KY, Berscheid BA, et al. Sensitivity and specificity of histamine PC20 determination in a random selection of young college students. J Allergy Clin Immunol 1992;89:23–30.
119. Carlsten C, Dimich-Ward H, Ferguson A, et al. Airway hyperresponsiveness to methacholine in 7-year-old children: sensitivity and specificity for pediatric allergist-diagnosed asthma. Pediatr Pulmonol 2011;46:175–8.
120. Hopp RJ, Bewtra AK, Nair NM, et al. Specificity and sensitivity of methacholine inhalation challenge in normal and asthmatic children. J Allergy Clin Immunol 1984;74:154–8.
121. Liem JJ, Kozyrskyj AL, Cockroft DW, et al. Diagnosing asthma in children: what is the role for methacholine bronchoprovocation testing? Pediatr Pulmonol 2008; 43:481–9.
122. Goldstein MF, Pacana SM, Dvorin DJ, et al. Retrospective analyses of methacholine inhalation challenges. Chest 1994;105:1082–8.
123. Nieminen MM. Unimodal distribution of bronchial hyperresponsiveness to methacholine in asthmatic patients. Chest 1992;102:1537–43.
124. Perpina M, Pellicer C, de Diego A, et al. Diagnostic value of the bronchial provocation test with methacholine in asthma. A Bayesian analysis approach. Chest 1993;104:149–54.
125. Sverrild A, Porsbjerg C, Thomsen SF, et al. Airway hyperresponsiveness to mannitol and methacholine and exhaled nitric oxide: a random-sample population study. J Allergy Clin Immunol 2010;126:952–8.
126. Goldstein MF, Veza BA, Dunsky EH, et al. Comparisons of peak diurnal expiratory flow variation, postbronchodilator FEV(1) responses, and methacholine inhalation challenges in the evaluation of suspected asthma. Chest 2001;119: 1001–10.
127. Sumino K, Sugar EA, Irvin CG, et al, American Lung Association Asthma Clinical Research Centers. Methacholine challenge test: diagnostic characteristics in asthmatic patients receiving controller medications. J Allergy Clin Immunol 2012;130:69–75.
128. Prieto L, Ferrer A, Domenech J, et al. Effect of challenge method on sensitivity, reactivity, and maximal response to methacholine. Ann Allergy Asthma Immunol 2006;97:175–81.
129. Wubbel C, Asmus MJ, Stevens G, et al. Methacholine challenge testing: comparison of the two American Thoracic Society-recommended methods. Chest 2004;125:453–8.
130. Siersted HC, Walker CM, O'Shaughnessy AD, et al. Comparison of two standardized methods of methacholine inhalation challenge in young adults. Eur Respir J 2000;15:181–4.
131. Cockcroft DW, Davis BE, Todd DC, et al. Methacholine challenge: comparison of two methods. Chest 2005;127(3):839–44.
132. Cockcroft DW. Methacholine challenge methods. Chest 2008;134:678–80.
133. Cockcroft DW, Davis BE. The bronchoprotective effect of inhaling methacholine by using total lung capacity inspirations has a marked influence on the interpretation of the test result. J Allergy Clin Immunol 2006;117:1244–8.

134. Coates AL, Wanger J, Cockcroft DW, et al. ERS technical standard on bronchial challenge testing: general considerations and performance of methacholine challenge tests. Eur Respir J 2017;49(5) [pii:1601526].

135. Dell SD, Bola SS, Foty R, et al. Provocative dose of methacholine causing a 20% drop in FEV1 should be used to interpret methacholine challenge tests with modern nebulizers. Ann Am Thorac Soc 2015;12:357–63.

136. Schulze J, Roswich M, Riemer C, et al. Methacholine challenge – comparison of an ATS protocol to a new rapid single concentration technique. Respir Med 2009;103:1898–903.

137. Cockcroft D, Davis B. Direct and indirect challenges in the clinical assessment of asthma. Ann Allergy Asthma Immunol 2009;103:363–70.

138. Porsbjerg C, Brannan JD, Anderson SD, et al. Relationship between airway responsiveness to mannitol and to methacholine and markers of airway inflammation, peak flow variability and quality of life in asthma patients. Clin Exp Allergy 2008;38:43–50.

139. Porsbjerg C, Backer V, Joos G, et al. Current and future use of the mannitol bronchial challenge in everyday clinical practice. Clin Respir J 2009;3:189–97.

140. Brannan JD, Koskela H, Anderson SD. Monitoring asthma therapy using indirect bronchial provocation tests. Clin Respir J 2007;1:3–15.

141. Kim MH, Song WJ, Kim TW, et al. Diagnostic properties of the methacholine and mannitol bronchial challenge tests: a comparison study. Respirology 2014;19: 852–6.

142. Leuppi JD, Salome CM, Jenkins CR, et al. Predictive markers of asthma exacerbations during stepwise dose reduction of inhaled corticosteroids. Am J Respir Crit Care Med 2001;163:406–12.

143. Koskela HO, Hyvarinen L, Brannan JD, et al. Sensitivity and validity of three bronchial provocation tests to demonstrate the effect of inhaled corticosteroids in asthma. Chest 2003;124:1341–9.

144. Singapuri A, McKenna S, Brightling CE, et al. Mannitol and AMP do not induce bronchoconstriction in eosinophilic bronchitis: further evidence for disassociation between airway inflammation and bronchial hyperresponsiveness. Respirology 2010;15:510–5.

145. Sue-Chu M, Brannan JD, Anderson SD, et al. Airway hyperresponsiveness to methacholine, adenosine5-monophosphate, mannitol, eucapnic voluntary hyperpnoea and field exercise challenge in elite cross country skiers. Br J Sports Med 2010;44:827–32.

146. Porsbjerg C, Rasmussen L, Thomsen SF, et al. Response to mannitol in asymptomatic subjects with airway hyper-responsiveness to methacholine. Clin Exp Allergy 2007;37:22–8.

147. Anderson SD, Brannan JD. Bronchial provocation testing: the future. Curr Opin Allergy Clin Immunol 2011;11(1):46–52.

148. Anderson SD. Indirect challenge tests: airway hyperresponsiveness in asthma: its measurement and clinical significance. Chest 2010;138(Suppl 2):25S–30S.

149. Anderton RC, Cu MT, Frith PA, et al. Bronchial responsiveness to inhaled histamine and exercise. J Allergy Clin Immunol 1979;63:315–20.

150. Holzer K, Anderson SD, Douglass J. Exercise in elite summer athletes: challenges for diagnosis. J Allergy Clin Immunol 2002;110:374–80.

151. Riedler J, Reade T, Dalton M, et al. Hypertonic saline challenge in an epidemiologic survey of asthma in children. Am J Respir Crit Care Med 1994;150: 1632–9.

152. O'Connor BJ, Ridge SM, Barnes PJ, et al. Greater effect of inhaled budesonide on adenosine 5'-monophosphate-induced than on sodium-metabisulfite-induced bronchoconstriction in asthma. Am Rev Respir Dis 1992;146:560–4.

153. Doull IJ, Sandall D, Smith S, et al. Differential inhibitory effect of regular inhaled corticosteroid on airway responsiveness to adenosine 5' monophosphate, methacholine, and bradykinin in symptomatic children with recurrent wheeze. Pediatr Pulmonol 1997;23:404–11.

154. Weersink EJ, Douma RR, Postma DS, et al. Flflucatisone propionate, salmeterol xinafoate, and their combination in the treatment of nocturnal asthma. Am J Respir Crit Care Med 1997;155:1241–6.

155. Reynolds CJ, Togias A, Proud D. Airways hyperresponsiveness to bradykinin and methacholine: effects of inhaled flucatisone. Clin Exp Allergy 2002;32:1174–9.

156. Church MK, Holgate ST, Hughes PJ. Adenosine inhibits and potentiates IgE-dependent histamine release from human basophils by an A2-receptor mediated mechanism. Br J Pharmacol 1983;80:719–26.

157. Hughes PJ, Holgate ST, Church MK. Adenosine inhibits and potentiates IgE-dependent histamine release from human lung mast cells by an A2- purinoceptor mediated mechanism. Biochem Pharmacol 1984;33:3847–52.

158. Peachell PT, Columbo M, Kagey-Sobotka A, et al. Adenosine potentiates mediator release from human lung mast cells. Am Rev Respir Dis 1988;138:1143–51.

159. Forsythe P, McGarvey LP, Heaney LG, et al. Adenosine induces histamine release from human bronchoalveolar lavage mast cells. Clin Sci 1999;96:349–55.

160. Fuller RW, Choudry NB, Eriksson G. Action of budesonide on asthmatic bronchial hyper-responsiveness: effects on directly and indirectly acting bronchoconstrictors. Chest 1991;100:670–4.

161. Vathenen AS, Knox AJ, Wisniewski A, et al. Effect of inhaled budesonide on bronchial reactivity to histamine, exercise, and eucapnic dry air in patients with asthma. Thorax 1991;46:811–6.

162. Rodwell LT, Anderson SD, Seale JP. Inhaled steroids modify bronchial responses to hyper-osmolar saline. Eur Respir J 1992;5:953–62.

163. du Toit JI, Anderson SD, Jenkins CR, et al. Airway responsiveness in asthma: bronchial challenge with histamine and 4.5% sodium chloride before and after budesonide. Allergy Asthma Proc 1997;18:7–14.

164. Global Initiative for Asthma (GINA). Global strategy for asthma management and prevention. 2018. Available at: https://ginasthma.org/2018-gina-report-global-strategy-for-asthma-management-and-prevention/.

165. National Asthma Education and Prevention Program. Expert panel report 3 (EPR-3): guidelines for the diagnosis and management of asthma, full report 2007. Bethesda (MD): US Department of Health and Human Services, National Institutes of Health, National Heart, Lung, and Blood Institute; 2007.

166. British Thoracic Society, Scottish Intercollegiate Guidelines Network. British guideline on the management of asthma. Thorax 2014;69(suppl 1):1–192.

167. van den Toorn LM, Overbeek SE, de Jongste JC, et al. Airway inflammation is present during clinical remission of atopic asthma. Am J Respir Crit Care Med 2001;164:2107–13.

168. Hanxiang N, Jiong Y, Yanwei C, et al. Persistent airway inflammation and bronchial hyperresponsiveness in patients with totally controlled asthma. Int J Clin Pract 2008;62(4):599–605.

169. Laprise C, Laviolette M, Boutet M, et al. Asymptomatic airway hyperresponsiveness: relationships with airway inflammation and remodelling. Eur Respir J 1999;14(1):63–73.

170. Saglani S, Lloyd CM. Novel concepts in airway inflammation and remodelling in asthma. Eur Respir J 2015;46(6):1796–804.
171. Deykin A, Lazarus SC, Fahy JV, et al. Sputum eosinophil counts predict asthma control after discontinuation of inhaled corticosteroids. J Allergy Clin Immunol 2005;115:720–7.
172. Dweik RA, Sorkness RL, Wenzel S, et al. Use of exhaled nitric oxide measurement to identify a reactive, at-risk phenotype among patients with asthma. Am J Respir Crit Care Med 2010;181:1033–41.
173. Anderson WJ, Short PM, Jabbal S, et al. Inhaled corticosteroid dose response in asthma: Should we measure inflammation? Ann Allergy Asthma Immunol 2017; 118(2):179–85.
174. Sont JK, Willems LN, Bel EH, et al. Clinical control and histopathologic outcome of asthma when using airway hyperresponsiveness as an additional guide to long-term treatment. Am J Respir Crit Care Med 1999;159(4 Pt 1):1043–51.
175. Nuijsink M, Hop WC, Sterk PJ, et al. Long-term asthma treatment guided by airway hyperresponsiveness in children: a randomised controlled trial. Eur Respir J 2007;30:457e66.
176. Nuijsink M, Vaessen-Verberne AA, Hop WC, et al. Long-term follow-up after two years of asthma treatment guided by airway responsiveness in children. Respir Med 2013;107(7):981–6.
177. Koenig SM, Murray JJ, Wolfe J, et al. Does measuring BHR add to guideline derived clinical measures in determining treatment for patients with persistent asthma? Respir Med 2008;102(5):665–73.
178. Brannan JD, Perry CP, Anderson SD. Mannitol test results in asthmatic adults receiving inhaled corticosteroids. J Allergy Clin Immunol 2013;131(3):906–7.
179. Prieto L, Ferrer A, Domenech J, et al. Predictive value of the response to inhaled adenosine 5'-monophosphate for reducing the dose of inhaled corticosteroids in asthma. J Investig Allergol Clin Immunol 2013;23(5):351–8.
180. Porsbjerg C, Lund TK, Pedersen L, et al. Inflammatory subtypes in asthma are related to airway hyperresponsiveness to mannitol and exhaled NO. J Asthma 2009;46(6):606–12.
181. Lipworth BJ, Short PM, Williamson PA, et al. A randomized primary care trial of steroid titration against mannitol in persistent asthma: STAMINA trial. Chest 2012;141(3):607–15.

Exhaled Nitric Oxide
An Update

Flavia C.L. Hoyte, MD[a],*, Lara M. Gross, MD[a,b],
Rohit K. Katial, MD[a]

KEYWORDS

- Exhaled nitric oxide • Allergic airway inflammation • Asthma • Exhaled NO • eNO
- FENO

KEY POINTS

- Fractional concentration of exhaled nitric oxide (FENO) is a noninvasive biomarker of allergic airway inflammation.
- FENO often correlates with eosinophilia, but is driven through different type 2 pathways.
- FENO can be a useful tool to aid in the diagnosis and management of respiratory disease, particularly asthma. However, guidelines on its use remain controversial.

Although originally described as endothelial-derived relaxing factor important in arterial tone, nitric oxide (NO) is now considered an important biomarker for respiratory disease.[1,2] Studies have confirmed that the fractional concentration of exhaled nitric oxide (FENO) is elevated in the airways of patients who have asthma compared with controls.[3–6] In addition, the level of FENO is well correlated with the presence and level of inflammation and decreases with glucocorticoid treatment.[6–8] Because this biomarker is noninvasively and easily collected, it has potential to be used not only as a diagnostic tool but also as a management tool for assessing severity, monitoring response to therapy, and gaining control of asthma symptoms. This article reviews the biology of NO and its role in respiratory disease.

BIOLOGY OF NITRIC OXIDE

NO, a gaseous molecule initially thought to be a deleterious component in environmental fumes, became the molecule of the year in 1992 and was found to be an

This article is an update of the previously published article on "Exhaled Nitric Oxide" in the August 2012 issue of the *Immunology and Allergy Clinics of North America*.
Disclosure Statement: No relevant disclosures.
[a] Division of Allergy and Immunology, National Jewish Health, 1400 Jackson Street, Denver, CO 80206, USA; [b] Division of Allergy and Clinical Immunology, Department of Medicine, University of Colorado, 13001 E 17th Place, Aurora, CO 80045, USA
* Corresponding author.
E-mail address: hoytef@njhealth.org

Immunol Allergy Clin N Am 38 (2018) 573–585
https://doi.org/10.1016/j.iac.2018.06.001
0889-8561/18/© 2018 Elsevier Inc. All rights reserved.

important signaling molecule in various biologic functions. This gas is abundant in the cardiovascular and respiratory systems.

NO and related compounds are generated from various resident and inflammatory cells in the human airway through the oxidation of L-arginine in the presence of a set of enzymes known as nitric oxide synthases (NOSs).[9,10] This process is both oxygen and NADPH dependent. NOSs are expressed in 3 isoforms that were originally referred to as either constitutive or inducible forms of NOS. The constitutive forms were classified according to their site of expression: neuronal or endothelial. However, these enzymes are now known to be expressed by a wide variety of pulmonary cells and are referred to as NOS1 and NOS3, respectively. The inducible form (iNOS or NOS2) is upregulated by proinflammatory cytokines and stimuli and is likely expressed continuously by human airway epithelial cells under normal conditions.[11,12]

In the lung, NOS1 is expressed in the NANC fibers and generates NO, which acts as a smooth muscle relaxer.[13,14] NOS3 has been found in pulmonary endothelium and bronchial and alveolar epithelium.[15,16] In the bronchial epithelium, NOS3 is thought to function primarily through regulating ciliary beat frequency.[17–19] Both NOS1 and NOS3 are corticosteroid resistant, and therefore, basal release of NO is not affected by steroids.[20,21]

NOS2 is a calcium/calmodulin–independent enzyme that is induced by tumor necrosis factor alpha, interferon gamma, interleukin-1β (IL-1β), viruses, bacteria, allergens, and environmental pollutants. In the respiratory tract, NOS2 has been reported to be expressed in epithelial cells, endothelium, airway and vascular smooth muscle, fibroblasts, mast cells, and neutrophils.[9] As opposed to constitutive Nitric Oxide Synthase (cNOS), NOS2 is glucocorticoid sensitive and, although some constitutive expression occurs in the airway epithelium, the level of pulmonary expression can be modulated. Once NOS2 is induced, the production of NO increases within several hours to nanomolar concentrations, levels that are significantly higher than basal levels resulting from cNOS NO production.

The role of NO in the lung includes neurotransmission, vasodilation, bronchial dilatation, and immune enhancement. However, NO has a paradoxic role in a disease such as asthma. In low concentrations, animal data support the bronchodilator nature of NO and the NANC-induced bronchodilation effect. However, at higher concentrations, NO seems to promote inflammation. Elevated exhaled NO values seen in disease states are suspected to be a result of overactivity of oxidative pathways, yielding proinflammatory cytokines and subsequent induction of NOS2 activity. The properties displayed by NO gas have allowed it to be measured in exhaled breath and to serve as a diagnostic and management tool for pulmonary disease.

MEASUREMENT AND INTERPRETATION

FENO is measured from a single breath exhalation. Measurement of FENO can be performed with either online techniques, where one exhales directly into an analyzer device and FENO is obtained immediately, or with offline techniques, where one exhales into a collection bag and the contents are later analyzed to determine the FENO. Measurements are more commonly performed online with real-time analyzers that measure NO with electrochemical sensors.[22] Online measurements are obtained with a single breath technique whereby a person inhales to total lung capacity and exhales at 50 mL/s (regulated through an inline resistance while providing feedback through a computer graphic interface) for approximately 6 seconds, the time required for the FENO levels to plateau. The maneuver is repeated twice at minimum to assure reproducibility. Exhalation against positive pressure causes the velum to close, which excludes upper respiratory NO from falsely raising the measurement of FENO.[23] Further information on technique is available in the American Thoracic Society (ATS)/European Respiratory Society (ERS) summary document.[24]

FENO levels are inversely proportional to the expiratory flow rate. High flow rates result in low FENO and, conversely, low flow rates yield higher FENO levels. Flow dependence is partially explained by the fact that FENO is partly derived from a diffusion-based process in the airways.[23,25] Because of this flow dependence, the ATS and the ERS adopted a standard for FENO measurements at 50 mL/s.

AIRFLOW MODELING

FENO is thought to provide insight into distal airway inflammation through a noninvasive route. Several investigators have described the sophisticated mathematical modeling, known as the 2-compartment model (alveolar and airway), allowing one to separately derive the relative contribution of the alveolar compartment to the overall NO production.[24–27] This model allows derivation of flow-independent parameters, such as airway wall NO concentration, airway diffusion factor, and alveolar NO concentration, which collectively determine the total exhaled NO production. The relationship between NO output and expiratory flow rate is used to derive the alveolar component. Applying this model to FENO measurements at multiple flow rates has helped to determine the alveolar and airway contributions. At fast flow rates (>50 mL/s), the alveolar contribution to the total NO value predominates, but at slower flow rates (<50 mL/s), airway diffusion predominates.[27]

NORMAL VALUES

There is ongoing variability regarding the normal reference range of FENO within adult and pediatric patient populations. Rather than using reference values, the current recommendation for interpreting FENO is to use clinical cut points. The current recommendation is that values <25 ppb (or <20 ppb for pediatrics) indicate a lack of allergic inflammation, whereas values >50 ppb (or >35 ppb for pediatrics) are likely to be consistent with allergic inflammation and responsive to corticosteroid treatment. Values ranging from 25 to 50 ppb (or 20–35 ppb for pediatrics) should be interpreted within the clinical context of each individual patient.[28]

The data attempting to identify normal levels of FENO are variable, and some study findings indicate different populations should have different cut points. Olin and colleagues[29] reported a median value of 15.8 ppb with an interquartile range of 11.9 to 21.4 ppb in 179 nonatopic healthy adults. The atopic asthmatic cohort showed a median value of 29.8 ppb with an interquartile range of 18.2 to 47.8 ppb.[29] Buchvald and colleagues[30] studied more than 400 children aged 4 to 17 years and found the mean FENO value to be 9.7 ppb. The upper end of the 95% confidence interval (CI) was age dependent, with a value of 15.7 ppb at age 4 and 25.2 ppb for adolescents, suggesting that perhaps there should be age-based FENO normal values.[30] A study by Yao and colleagues[31] also supported the idea of age-based FENO normal values, because they found that FENO increased by an average of 7.4% per year in children. The effect of age on FENO is limited to children, because FENO increases with age until adulthood and then stabilizes.[32,33]

Another study in pediatric patients demonstrated that in addition to age, race and height were important factors in determining baseline FENO values.[34] Olivieri and colleagues[35] measured FENO levels in more than 200 non-smoking adults. Men were found to have levels ranging from 2.6 to 28.8 ppb, and women had levels ranging from 1.6 to 21.5 ppb. In another study by Travers and colleagues,[36] men consistently had higher levels of FENO than women. The difference between men and women suggests a possible need to have gender-specific normal values. However, a study by Olin and colleagues[37] found that age and height affected FENO, but gender did not. Olin and colleagues[38] also published FENO values from a random general population sample and found the median value to be 16 ppb, with the 25th to 75th percentiles being 11 and 22.3 ppb, respectively. Height, age, atopy, report of asthma symptoms in the past month, and reported use of inhaled steroids were positively associated with FENO, whereas current smokers had lower values of FENO. In general, both short-term and chronic smoking cause decreased FENO levels, but FENO levels are usually still elevated in smoking patients who have asthma.[5,38–40] Gender was not associated with FENO in this study, although other studies have shown FENO to be higher in men than women.[38,41]

The most recent ATS guidelines on interpreting FENO suggest evaluating changes in an individual's FENO from personal baseline in addition to using generalized cut points. Based on studies evaluating the utility of FENO in guiding dose adjustment of inhaled corticosteroids, an increase or decrease in FENO greater than 20% for levels greater than 50 ppb (or a difference greater than 10 ppb for levels <50 ppb) is significant.[28]

FACTORS ASSOCIATED WITH ELEVATED NITRIC OXIDE
Allergic and Eosinophilic Inflammation

Allergic and eosinophilic inflammation are central hallmarks of asthma. Studies have confirmed a strong, although not always absolute, correlation between FENO and eosinophilia in induced sputum,[42,43] bronchoalveolar lavage,[44] and tissue.[45–47] Berry and colleagues[48] demonstrated that an FENO of 36 ppb had a sensitivity of 78% and a specificity of 72% for sputum eosinophils greater than 3%. The meta-analysis of Korevaar and colleagues[49] found that FENO had a sensitivity of 66% and a specificity of 76% for detecting sputum eosinophils of 3% or greater in adults. Thus, although FENO can be used as a noninvasive surrogate for sputum eosinophils, this may result in several false positives or negatives.[49] Payne and colleagues[46] obtained endobronchial biopsies in asthmatic children aged 6 to 17 years treated with prednisolone. Those who had persistent symptoms and a raised eosinophil score showed higher FENO levels.[46,50] Similarly, in a study of 29 children with asthma and nonasthmatic controls, Warke and colleagues[44] showed that FENO was positively correlated with BAL eosinophil levels.

Allergenic exposures induce T-helper 2 cell (Th2)-mediated inflammation, leading to increased levels of IL-4, IL-5, and IL-13.[51] In addition, type 2 innate lymphoid cells (ILC2) can be stimulated by allergenic or nonallergenic stimuli, such as alarmin cytokines like IL-33, to release IL-5 and IL-13.[51,52] IL-4 and IL-13 seem to drive FENO, whereas IL-5 drives eosinophilia. Because these cytokines can often increase or decrease at the same time for a given individual, eosinophils and FENO can often increase or decrease in parallel. The correlation is not absolute, however, because eosinophilia and FENO are driven by different cytokines that are produced by various cells, and the relative production of these cytokines will help determine the trajectory of each biomarker.

Recent studies of biologic agents in asthma have helped elucidate the different mechanisms driving allergic and eosinophilic inflammation and their relationship to FENO. In the DREAM study looking at the exacerbation-reducing effect of mepolizumab, a monoclonal antibody to IL-5, subjects were required to meet 1 of 4 criteria that could possibly represent an eosinophilic phenotype: elevated FENO ≥50 ppb, blood eosinophilia $\geq$300, sputum eosinophilia $\geq$3%, or asthma deterioration with a <25% decrease in Inhaled corticosteroid (ICS) and oral corticosteroid (OCS) dose. The study found that although FENO and blood eosinophils correlated with sputum eosinophils, baseline blood eosinophils were closely associated with a response to mepolizumab, whereas baseline FENO was not.[53] A study evaluating the efficacy of lebrikizumab, an anti-IL-13 antibody, for asthma found that treatment with lebrikizumab decreased FENO levels.[54] Similarly, the use of dupilumab, a monoclonal antibody that inhibits IL-4 and IL-13, appears to decrease FENO. In a pilot study looking at dupilumab's ability to reduce "induced exacerbations" when ICS and Long acting beta-agonist (LABA) were weaned, FENO levels decreased and remained decreased even with a weaning of ICS therapy. There were no significant changes in eosinophil levels in the treatment or placebo group.[55] A larger, more recent study of dupilumab in adult asthmatics demonstrated a decrease in FENO in both those with elevated eosinophils and those with low or normal eosinophils at baseline.[56]

Although these varied results to the biologics may seem inconsistent initially, understanding the signaling pathway for FENO sheds light on these. Because iNOS is activated by STAT1 and STAT6, upregulation of STAT6 through upregulation of IL-4 and IL-13 would in turn be associated with higher FENO levels. On the other hand, IL-5 upregulates STAT5, which does not have an effect on iNOS or FENO levels. Understanding this pathway further supports the idea that FENO is not a surrogate marker for sputum eosinophils but rather an often parallel marker of airway inflammation.

Glucocorticoid Responsiveness

The correlation of FENO with allergic and eosinophilic inflammation suggests that FENO is also useful to predict steroid responsiveness. In 2003, the US Food and Drug Administration approved the Aerocrine AB (Stockholm, Sweden) FENO monitoring system for clinical application in patients who have asthma. The labeling of this device was restricted to monitoring the response to anti-inflammatory medications, as an adjunct to established clinical and laboratory assessments, in individuals aged 4 to 65.[57]

Little and colleagues[58] studied the use of FENO as a marker for response to oral glucocorticoids in adults with stable asthma and found that the clinical benefit of oral steroids was greatest in those showing elevated baseline FENO levels. In a study of severe, therapy-resistant pediatric asthma patients, FENO, along with ACT score, forced expiratory volume in 1 second (FEV1), and sputum eosinophils, was examined to predict systemic steroid responsiveness.[59] Smith and colleagues[60] found similar results in a study of 52 steroid-naive adults with chronic respiratory symptoms who received 4 weeks of inhaled fluticasone therapy. The response to ICS as assessed through symptoms and spirometry was greatest in the third of subjects whose FENO was greater than 47 ppb. In the absence of a high FENO, the response to steroids was less likely.[60] Similarly, Szefler and colleagues[61] showed that asthmatic children who had high FENO values as well as elevation in other allergic markers (peripheral eosinophils, total immunoglobulin E, and eosinophil cationic protein) were more likely to respond to ICS than those who had lower FENO and other allergic biomarkers. Thus, higher FENO levels appear to predict steroid responsiveness, particularly in allergic asthma.

Similarly, several studies have supported the use of FENO to adjust ICS dose. A study by Pijnenburg and colleagues[62] evaluated 85 children who had asthma. Using 30 ppb as the threshold above which therapy would be increased, a significant reduction in bronchial hyperresponsiveness was seen in the FENO group, with a concomitant reduction in exacerbations requiring oral steroid use. Katsara and colleagues[63] assessed compliance using FENO and a data logger attached to a pressurized meter dose inhaler. This study showed a tendency toward increased FENO with poor compliance. Although these studies do not conclusively prove cause and effect, they suggest the usefulness of FENO as a noninvasive marker in the clinical setting to adjust ICS dose and to monitor patient compliance.

Respiratory Infections

Exhaled NO is increased in association with some viral infections but not with bacterial infections.[64,65] A study investigating the presence of rhinovirus in nasopharyngeal aspirate from asymptomatic stable asthmatic patients and healthy controls demonstrated rhinovirus prevalence of 4.5% in asthmatics versus 0.9% in controls. The asthmatics who were positive for rhinovirus had higher FENOs than their rhinovirus-negative counterparts, although this did not reach significance.

Unlike infections with rhinovirus, infections with respiratory syncytial virus appear to result in a reduction in NO formation. The difference has been hypothesized to be due to the ability of some viruses to induce iNOS expression. The pathway of this induction is unclear but may be linked to activation of STAT-1 via interferons. In addition, viruses such as rhinovirus and influenza A, are thought to induce ILC2s and IL-33 production, leading to increased production of Th2 cytokines, as discussed earlier, which could account for the increase in FENO.[66]

CLINICAL USE
Asthma

Because FENO has been positively correlated with the presence of airway eosinophilia and allergic inflammation, it may be useful as an asthma diagnostic test to assess underlying inflammation. An official ATS clinical practice guideline published in 2011 based on a committee of FENO experts recommended the use of FENO in diagnosing eosinophilic airway inflammation and in determining steroid responsiveness; however, the 2013 ATS/ERS severe asthma guidelines do not recommend using FENO to guide treatment of severe asthma. Notably, this recommendation is conditional with very low-quality evidence.[28,67] Similarly, the 2017 Global Initiative for Asthma guidelines do not support the use of FENO for making or excluding a diagnosis of asthma, and they do not recommend using FENO to help decide whether or not to initiate ICS therapy.[68]

Dupont and colleagues[69] studied steroid-naive subjects without a diagnosis of asthma who had symptoms suggestive of asthma. Of the 240 people, 160 had asthma based on post–bronchodilator reversibility in FEV1. In this study, FENO levels were found to have a sensitivity and specificity of 85% and 90%, respectively. Schneider and colleagues[70] used statistical modeling of data from 26 studies to conclude that when the pretest probability is at least 30%, FENO greater than 50 ppb has a positive predictive value of 0.76 (95% CI: 0.29–0.96) for diagnosing asthma. Smith and colleagues[71] compared conventional diagnostic tests for asthma (bronchial hyperreactivity or beta-agonist reversibility) with FENO and induced sputum markers. Of the 47 subjects with symptoms suggesting asthma, 17 were ultimately diagnosed using the conventional diagnostic tests. In these individuals, FENO had a sensitivity and specificity of 88% and 79%, respectively.[71]

FENO can also be helpful in diagnosing cough-variant asthma in patients with chronic cough. A meta-analysis of 15 studies by Song and colleagues[41] found that in a population with chronic cough, FENO had a sensitivity of 72% and a specificity of 85% for diagnosing cough-variant asthma, suggesting FENO could be a helpful rule-in test for diagnosing cough-variant asthma. Of note, many of the studies supporting the use of FENO for diagnosing asthma were conducted in individuals without a prior respiratory diagnosis, which presumably means their disease was mild.

A meta-analysis of 43 studies evaluating the diagnostic accuracy of FENO for asthma concluded that FENO was a more accurate diagnostic tool in children than in adults. The investigators note that in the pediatric population overdiagnosis of asthma is much more common than underdiagnosis.[72]

Malinovschi and colleagues[73] studied FENO as a marker for local inflammation and blood eosinophils as a marker for systemic inflammation to examine their relationship with wheeze, asthma diagnosis, asthma exacerbation, and emergency department (ED) visits. In a population of more than 12,000 children and adults, they found that there was a statistically significant but weak correlation between FENO and blood eosinophils. Both FENO and blood eosinophils correlated positively with asthma, wheeze, and asthma attacks, but only elevated blood eosinophils correlated with ED visits. The investigators hypothesized that the association between exacerbation in patients with severe asthma and eosinophils may be due to rhinovirus-triggered exacerbations, also causing an increase in eosinophils through the ILC2 pathway. FENO and blood eosinophils were found to have an additive value in predicting asthma and wheeze. In another study of FENO and asthma control, Malinovschi and colleagues[73,74] investigated the utility of using FENO and blood eosinophilia to predict bronchial hyperreactivity and uncontrolled asthma in asthmatics aged 10 to 35. They found that using both FENO and blood eosinophils predicted poor asthma control better than using blood eosinophils or FENO alone.

To correlate FENO values and asthma control, Jatakanon and colleagues[75] used a steroid reduction model. They evaluated 15 asthma patients twice weekly over 8 weeks after inhaled steroid reduction. Elevated FENO levels significantly correlated with decreased airway function, decreased FEV1, and increased frequency of beta-agonist use. In another study, asthma control was assessed in 30 patients based on conventional measures of symptoms and lung function. FENO correlated with both asthma control and severity level.[76]

Several studies have evaluated the use of FENO to adjust treatment as well as to assess asthma control. Meyts and colleagues[77] conducted an office-based evaluation of asthma control in 73 children aged 5 to 18 years. Three levels of control (good, acceptable, and insufficient) were determined based on frequency of beta-agonist use, day and nighttime symptoms, and spirometry. The subjects determined to have insufficiently controlled disease had the highest median levels of FENO (median 28 ppb).[77]

Similar to other studies,[78,79] a prospective trial by Smith and colleagues[80] evaluated the usefulness of repeat measurements of FENO to guide therapy as compared with a guideline-based management strategy. The FENO group experienced a 46% reduction in the number of exacerbations, but based on a predefined cutoff for analysis, this reduction did not reach statistical significance. However, a statistically significant reduction did occur in mean ICS use over 12 months for the group managed using FENO measurements.[80] In a study of asthma in pregnancy, an FENO-guided treatment algorithm resulted in fewer exacerbations than symptom-guided treatment.[81] Powell and colleagues[81] demonstrated that using FENO to guide ICS dose, in addition to using symptoms to guide LABA use, reduced asthma exacerbations when compared with medication dosing guided by symptoms alone. In addition, the FENO group required significantly less Short acting beta-agonist (SABA) use, and the mean daily ICS dose of those in the FENO-guided group was less than the symptom-guided group.

In contrast, Szefler and colleagues[82] demonstrated that adjusting treatment based on FENO levels in an inner-city asthmatic pediatric population resulted in higher doses of inhaled corticosteroids compared with management based on symptoms alone. Moreover, there is a small fraction of asthmatic patients in whom FENO fails to improve despite treatment with corticosteroids.[83] In atopic children with asthma, persistently elevated FENO may be due to ongoing allergen exposure and related to the level of allergic sensitization.[84] The negative results in Szefler's study may have been due to a combination of ongoing allergen exposure in the inner-city cohort as well as to the fact that their asthma and FENO levels were optimized before randomization, leading to difficulty detecting a difference when using symptoms as an outcome measure. Despite these findings, most studies to date support the concept that using a measure of inflammation, such as FENO, to help guide therapy may lead to more effective disease management, gauged by minimizing exacerbations and optimizing medication use.

Chronic Obstructive Pulmonary Disease

Because of its usefulness in diagnosing and assessing inflammation in asthma, FENO as a tool for diagnosing and monitoring chronic obstructive pulmonary disease (COPD) was investigated. FENO has not been found to be elevated in stable COPD,[85,86] likely due to the prevalence of cigarette smoking and predominance of neutrophilic inflammation seen in these patients.[86] A small but detectable difference is seen in patients who have COPD and are current smokers compared with COPD patients who are ex-smokers or those who have never smoked.[87] Obtaining an FENO level may have a role in patients who have unstable COPD and those experiencing COPD exacerbations. These patients were found to have elevated FENO levels when compared with patients who had stable COPD (both smokers and ex-smokers).[88] There may also be a role for FENO in assessing patients with asthma-COPD overlap.

SUMMARY

Before the use of FENO, direct assessment of airway inflammation was limited to invasive techniques. Continued understanding and correlations of FENO measurements will likely continue to complement conventional diagnostic and assessment tools for inflammatory lung disease. Because the technique is noninvasive, it has gained popularity and is becoming a more common tool used not only for initial diagnosis but also for routine assessment of disease severity, response to treatment, and compliance. Furthermore, monitoring of FENO can help characterize various asthma phenotypes within the asthma syndrome and guide the appropriate use of inhaled corticosteroids as well as potentially biologics. Although a precise normal has yet to be defined, strong data exist for high positive and negative predictive values for diagnosing and treating asthma at both ends of the spectrum of FENO values. High FENO values (>50 ppb) suggest poor control, the presence of persistent inflammation, and a need for increased anti-inflammatory treatment. Low values (<25 ppb) suggest low levels of inflammation and may allow for anti-inflammatory treatment withdrawal. Currently, FENO serves as a complementary tool in managing patients who have asthma and other inflammatory diseases in addition to conventional measures of symptom control and response to therapy.

REFERENCES

1. Palmer RMJ, Ferrige AG, Moncada SA. Nitric oxide release accounts for the biological activity of endothelium-derived relaxing factor. Nature 1987;327:524–6.

2. Gustafsson LE, Leone AM, Persson MG, et al. Endogenous nitric oxide is present in the exhaled air of rabbits, guinea pigs and humans. Biochem Biophys Res Commun 1991;181(2):852–7.

3. Alving K, Weitzberg E, Lundberg JM. Increased amount of nitric oxide in exhaled air of asthmatics. Eur Respir J 1993;6(9):1368.

4. Kharitonov SA, Yates D, Robbins RA, et al. Increased nitric oxide in exhaled air of asthmatic patients. Lancet 1994;343(8890):133–5.

5. Persson MG, Gustafsson LE, Zetterström O, et al. Single-breath nitric oxide measurements in asthmatic patients and smokers. Lancet 1994;343(8890):146–7.

6. Yates DH, Kharitonov SA, Robbins RA, et al. Effect of a nitric oxide synthase inhibitor and a glucocorticosteroid on exhaled nitric oxide. Am J Respir Crit Care Med 1995;152(3):892–6.

7. Kharitonov SA, Yates DH, Barnes PJ. Inhaled glucocorticoids decrease nitric oxide in exhaled air of asthmatic patients. Am J Respir Crit Care Med 1996;153(1):454–7.

8. Massaro AF, Gaston B, Kita D, et al. Expired nitric oxide levels during treatment of acute asthma. Am J Respir Crit Care Med 1995;152(2):800–3.

9. Ricciardolo FLM, Sterk PJ, Gaston B, et al. Nitric oxide in health and disease of the respiratory system. Physiol Rev 2004;84(3):731–65.

10. Förstermann U, Schmidt HHHW, Pollock JS, et al. Isoforms of nitric oxide synthase Characterization and purification from different cell types. Biochem Pharmacol 1991;42(10):1849–57.

11. Guo FH, De Raeve HR, Rice TW, et al. Continuous nitric oxide synthesis by inducible nitric oxide synthase in normal human airway epithelium in vivo. Proc Natl Acad Sci U S A 1995;92(17):7809–13.

12. Fischer A, Folkerts G, Geppetti P, et al. Mediators of asthma: nitric oxide. Pulm Pharmacol Ther 2002;15(2):73–81.

13. Belvisi MG, Stretton CD, Yacoub M, et al. Nitric oxide is the endogenous neurotransmitter of bronchodilator nerves in humans. Eur J Pharmacol 1992;210(2):221–2.

14. Li CG, Rand MJ. Evidence that part of the NANC relaxant response of guinea-pig trachea to electrical field stimulation is mediated by nitric oxide. Br J Pharmacol 1991;102(1):91–4.

15. Shaul PW, North AJ, Wu LC, et al. Endothelial nitric oxide synthase is expressed in cultured human bronchiolar epithelium. J Clin Invest 1994;94(6):2231–6.

16. Pechkovsky DV, Zissel G, Goldmann T, et al. Pattern of NOS2 and NOS3 mRNA expression in human A549 cells and primary cultured AEC II. Am J Physiol Lung Cell Mol Physiol 2002;282(4):L684–92.

17. Li D, Shirakami G, Zhan X, et al. Regulation of ciliary beat frequency by the nitric oxide-cyclic guanosine monophosphate signaling pathway in rat airway epithelial cells. Am J Respir Cell Mol Biol 2000;23(2):175–81.

18. Gertsberg I, Hellman V, Fainshtein M, et al. Intracellular Ca2+ regulates the phosphorylation and the dephosphorylation of ciliary proteins via the NO pathway. J Gen Physiol 2004;124(5):527–40.

19. Jain B, Rubinstein I, Robbins RA, et al. Modulation of airway epithelial cell ciliary beat frequency by nitric oxide. Biochem Biophys Res Commun 1993;191(1):83–8.

20. Di Rosa M, Radomski M, Carnuccio R, et al. Glucocorticoids inhibit the induction of nitric oxide synthase in macrophages. Biochem Biophys Res Commun 1990;172(3):1246–52.

21. Radomski MW, Palmer RM, Moncada S. Glucocorticoids inhibit the expression of an inducible, but not the constitutive, nitric oxide synthase in vascular endothelial cells. Proc Natl Acad Sci U S A 1990;87(24):10043–7.

22. Maniscalco M, Vitale C, Vatrella A, et al. Fractional exhaled nitric oxide-measuring devices: technology update. Med Devices (Auckl) 2016;9:151–60.

23. Silkoff PE, McClean PA, Slutsky AS, et al. Marked flow-dependence of exhaled nitric oxide using a new technique to exclude nasal nitric oxide. Am J Respir Crit Care Med 1997;155(1):260–7.

24. ATS/ERS recommendations for standardized procedures for the online and offline measurement of exhaled lower respiratory nitric oxide and nasal nitric oxide, 2005. Am J Respir Crit Care Med 2005;171(8):912–30.

25. Silkoff PE, Sylvester JT, Zamel N, et al. Airway nitric oxide diffusion in asthma: Role in pulmonary function and bronchial responsiveness. Am J Respir Crit Care Med 2000;161(4 Pt 1):1218–28.

26. George SC, Hogman M, Permutt S, et al. Modeling pulmonary nitric oxide exchange. J Appl Physiol (1985) 2004;96(3):831–9.

27. Tsoukias NM, George SC. A two-compartment model of pulmonary nitric oxide exchange dynamics. J Appl Physiol (1985) 1998;85(2):653–66.

28. Dweik RA, Boggs PB, Erzurum SC, et al. An official ATS clinical practice guideline: interpretation of exhaled nitric oxide levels (FENO) for clinical applications. Am J Respir Crit Care Med 2011;184(5):602–15.

29. Olin AC, Alving K, Toren K. Exhaled nitric oxide: relation to sensitization and respiratory symptoms. Clin Exp Allergy 2004;34(2):221–6.

30. Buchvald F, Baraldi E, Carraro S, et al. Measurements of exhaled nitric oxide in healthy subjects age 4 to 17 years. J Allergy Clin Immunol 2005;115(6):1130–6.

31. Yao TC, Ou LS, Lee WI, et al. Exhaled nitric oxide discriminates children with and without allergic sensitization in a population-based study. Clin Exp Allergy 2011; 41(4):556–64.

32. Franklin PJ, Taplin R, Stick SM. A community study of exhaled nitric oxide in healthy children. Am J Respir Crit Care Med 1999;159(1):69–73.

33. Kissoon N, Duckworth LJ, Blake KV, et al. Exhaled nitric oxide concentrations: online versus offline values in healthy children. Pediatr Pulmonol 2002;33(4):283–92.

34. Kovesi T, Kulka R, Dales R. Exhaled nitric oxide concentration is affected by age, height, and race in healthy 9- to 12-year-old children. Chest 2008;133(1):169–75.

35. Olivieri M, Malerba M, Talamini G, et al. Reference values for exhaled nitric oxide in the general population. Chest 2008;133(3):831–2.

36. Travers J, Marsh S, Aldington S, et al. Reference ranges for exhaled nitric oxide derived from a random community survey of adults. Am J Respir Crit Care Med 2007;176(3):238–42.

37. Olin AC, Bake B, Toren K. Fraction of exhaled nitric oxide at 50 mL/s: reference values for adult lifelong never-smokers. Chest 2007;131(6):1852–6.

38. Olin AC, Rosengren A, Thelle DS, et al. Height, age, and atopy are associated with fraction of exhaled nitric oxide in a large adult general population sample. Chest 2006;130(5):1319–25.

39. Chambers DC, Tunnicliffe WS, Ayres JG. Acute inhalation of cigarette smoke increases lower respiratory tract nitric oxide concentrations. Thorax 1998;53(8): 677–9.

40. Horvath I, Donnelly LE, Kiss A, et al. Exhaled nitric oxide and hydrogen peroxide concentrations in asthmatic smokers. Respiration 2004;71(5):463–8.

41. Song WJ, Kim HJ, Shim JS, et al. Diagnostic accuracy of fractional exhaled nitric oxide measurement in predicting cough-variant asthma and eosinophilic

bronchitis in adults with chronic cough: a systematic review and meta-analysis. J Allergy Clin Immunol 2017;140(3):701–9.

42. Berlyne GS, Parameswaran K, Kamada D, et al. A comparison of exhaled nitric oxide and induced sputum as markers of airway inflammation. J Allergy Clin Immunol 2000;106(4):638–44.

43. Jatakanon A, Lim S, Kharitonov SA, et al. Correlation between exhaled nitric oxide, sputum eosinophils, and methacholine responsiveness in patients with mild asthma. Thorax 1998;53(2):91–5.

44. Warke TJ, Fitch PS, Brown V, et al. Exhaled nitric oxide correlates with airway eosinophils in childhood asthma. Thorax 2002;57(5):383–7.

45. Brightling CE, Symon FA, Birring SS, et al. Comparison of airway immunopathology of eosinophilic bronchitis and asthma. Thorax 2003;58(6):528–32.

46. Payne DN, Adcock IM, Wilson NM, et al. Relationship between exhaled nitric oxide and mucosal eosinophilic inflammation in children with difficult asthma, after treatment with oral prednisolone. Am J Respir Crit Care Med 2001;164(8 Pt 1): 1376–81.

47. van den Toorn LM, Overbeek SE, de Jongste JC, et al. Airway inflammation is present during clinical remission of atopic asthma. Am J Respir Crit Care Med 2001; 164(11):2107–13.

48. Berry MA, Shaw DE, Green RH, et al. The use of exhaled nitric oxide concentration to identify eosinophilic airway inflammation: an observational study in adults with asthma. Clin Exp Allergy 2005;35(9):1175–9.

49. Korevaar DA, Westerhof GA, Wang J, et al. Diagnostic accuracy of minimally invasive markers for detection of airway eosinophilia in asthma: a systematic review and meta-analysis. Lancet Respir Med 2015;3(4):290–300.

50. Bove PF, van der Vliet A. Nitric oxide and reactive nitrogen species in airway epithelial signaling and inflammation. Free Radic Biol Med 2006;41(4):515–27.

51. Chen R, Smith SG, Salter B, et al. Allergen-induced increases in sputum levels of group 2 innate lymphoid cells in subjects with asthma. Am J Respir Crit Care Med 2017;196(6):700–12.

52. Hirose K, Iwata A, Tamachi T, et al. Allergic airway inflammation: key players beyond the Th2 cell pathway. Immunol Rev 2017;278(1):145–61.

53. Pavord ID, Korn S, Howarth P, et al. Mepolizumab for severe eosinophilic asthma (DREAM): a multicentre, double-blind, placebo-controlled trial. Lancet 2012; 380(9842):651–9.

54. Corren J, Lemanske RF, Hanania NA, et al. Lebrikizumab treatment in adults with asthma. N Engl J Med 2011;365(12):1088–98.

55. Wenzel S, Ford L, Pearlman D, et al. Dupilumab in persistent asthma with elevated eosinophil levels. N Engl J Med 2013;368(26):2455–66.

56. Wenzel S, Castro M, Corren J, et al. Dupilumab efficacy and safety in adults with uncontrolled persistent asthma despite use of medium-to-high-dose inhaled corticosteroids plus a long-acting beta2 agonist: a randomised double-blind placebo-controlled pivotal phase 2b dose-ranging trial. Lancet 2016;388(10039): 31–44.

57. Silkoff PE, Carlson M, Bourke T, et al. The Aerocrine exhaled nitric oxide monitoring system NIOX is cleared by the US Food and Drug Administration for monitoring therapy in asthma. J Allergy Clin Immunol 2004;114(5):1241–56.

58. Little SA, Chalmers GW, MacLeod KJ, et al. Non-invasive markers of airway inflammation as predictors of oral steroid responsiveness in asthma. Thorax 2000;55(3):232–4.

59. Bossley CJ, Fleming L, Ullmann N, et al. Assessment of corticosteroid response in pediatric patients with severe asthma by using a multidomain approach. J Allergy Clin Immunol 2016;138(2):413–20.e6.

60. Smith AD, Cowan JO, Brassett KP, et al. Exhaled nitric oxide: a predictor of steroid response. Am J Respir Crit Care Med 2005;172(4):453–9.

61. Szefler SJ, Phillips BR, Martinez FD, et al. Characterization of within-subject responses to fluticasone and montelukast in childhood asthma. J Allergy Clin Immunol 2005;115(2):233–42.

62. Pijnenburg MW, Bakker EM, Hop WC, et al. Titrating steroids on exhaled nitric oxide in children with asthma: a randomized controlled trial. Am J Respir Crit Care Med 2005;172(7):831–6.

63. Katsara M, Donnelly D, Iqbal S, et al. Relationship between exhaled nitric oxide levels and compliance with inhaled corticosteroids in asthmatic children. Respir Med 2006;100(9):1512–7.

64. Kharitonov SA, Yates D, Barnes PJ. Increased nitric oxide in exhaled air of normal human subjects with upper respiratory tract infections. Eur Respir J 1995;8(2):295–7.

65. Carraro S, Andreola B, Alinovi R, et al. Exhaled leukotriene B4 in children with community acquired pneumonia. Pediatr Pulmonol 2008;43(10):982–6.

66. Papi A, Bellettato CM, Braccioni F, et al. Infections and airway inflammation in chronic obstructive pulmonary disease severe exacerbations. Am J Respir Crit Care Med 2006;173(10):1114–21.

67. Chung KF, Wenzel SE, Brozek JL, et al. International ERS/ATS guidelines on definition, evaluation and treatment of severe asthma. Eur Respir J 2014;43(2):343–73.

68. Global Initiative for Asthma. Global strategy for asthma management and prevention. 2017 Available at: https://ginasthma.org/2018-gina-report-global-strategy-for-asthma-management-and-prevention/.

69. Dupont LJ, Demedts MG, Verleden GM. Prospective evaluation of the validity of exhaled nitric oxide for the diagnosis of asthma. Chest 2003;123(3):751–6.

70. Schneider A, Linde K, Reitsma JB, et al. A novel statistical model for analyzing data of a systematic review generates optimal cutoff values for fractional exhaled nitric oxide for asthma diagnosis. J Clin Epidemiol 2017;92:69–78.

71. Smith AD, Cowan JO, Filsell S, et al. Diagnosing asthma: comparisons between exhaled nitric oxide measurements and conventional tests. Am J Respir Crit Care Med 2004;169(4):473–8.

72. Wang Z, Pianosi PT, Keogh KA, et al. The diagnostic accuracy of fractional exhaled nitric oxide testing in asthma: a systematic review and meta-analyses. Mayo Clin Proc 2017;93(2):191–8.

73. Malinovschi A, Fonseca JA, Jacinto T, et al. Exhaled nitric oxide levels and blood eosinophil counts independently associate with wheeze and asthma events in National Health and Nutrition Examination Survey subjects. J Allergy Clin Immunol 2013;132(4):821–7.e1-5.

74. Malinovschi A, Janson C, Borres M, et al. Simultaneously increased fraction of exhaled nitric oxide levels and blood eosinophil counts relate to increased asthma morbidity. J Allergy Clin Immunol 2016;138(5):1301–8.e2.

75. Jatakanon A, Lim S, Barnes PJ. Changes in sputum eosinophils predict loss of asthma control. Am J Respir Crit Care Med 2000;161(1):64–72.

76. Delgado-Corcoran C, Kissoon N, Murphy SP, et al. Exhaled nitric oxide reflects asthma severity and asthma control. Pediatr Crit Care Med 2004;5(1):48–52.

77. Meyts I, Proesmans M, De Boeck K. Exhaled nitric oxide corresponds with office evaluation of asthma control. Pediatr Pulmonol 2003;36(4):283–9.
78. Sont JK, Willems LN, Bel EH, et al. Clinical control and histopathologic outcome of asthma when using airway hyperresponsiveness as an additional guide to long-term treatment. The AMPUL Study Group. Am J Respir Crit Care Med 1999;159(4 Pt 1):1043–51.
79. Green RH, Brightling CE, Woltmann G, et al. Analysis of induced sputum in adults with asthma: identification of subgroup with isolated sputum neutrophilia and poor response to inhaled corticosteroids. Thorax 2002;57(10):875–9.
80. Smith AD, Cowan JO, Brassett KP, et al. Use of exhaled nitric oxide measurements to guide treatment in chronic asthma. N Engl J Med 2005;352(21): 2163–73.
81. Powell H, Murphy VE, Taylor DR, et al. Management of asthma in pregnancy guided by measurement of fraction of exhaled nitric oxide: a double-blind, randomised controlled trial. Lancet 2011;378(9795):983–90.
82. Szefler SJ, Mitchell H, Sorkness CA, et al. Management of asthma based on exhaled nitric oxide in addition to guideline-based treatment for inner-city adolescents and young adults: a randomised controlled trial. Lancet 2008;372(9643): 1065–72.
83. Pijnenburg MW, Bakker EM, Lever S, et al. High fractional concentration of nitric oxide in exhaled air despite steroid treatment in asthmatic children. Clin Exp Allergy 2005;35(7):920–5.
84. Buchvald F, Eiberg H, Bisgaard H. Heterogeneity of FeNO response to inhaled steroid in asthmatic children. Clin Exp Allergy 2003;33(12):1735–40.
85. Robbins RA, Floreani AA, Von Essen SG, et al. Measurement of exhaled nitric oxide by three different techniques. Am J Respir Crit Care Med 1996;153(5): 1631–5.
86. Corradi M, Majori M, Cacciani GC, et al. Increased exhaled nitric oxide in patients with stable chronic obstructive pulmonary disease. Thorax 1999;54(7):572–5.
87. Bhowmik A, Seemungal TA, Donaldson GC, et al. Effects of exacerbations and seasonality on exhaled nitric oxide in COPD. Eur Respir J 2005;26(6):1009–15.
88. Maziak W, Loukides S, Culpitt S, et al. Exhaled nitric oxide in chronic obstructive pulmonary disease. Am J Respir Crit Care Med 1998;157(3 Pt 1):998–1002.

Immunoglobulin E as a Biomarker in Asthma

Niharika Rath, MD[a], Nikita Raje, MD[a], Lanny Rosenwasser, MD[b],*

KEYWORDS

- IgE • Asthma • Biomarker • Biotherapy

KEY POINTS

- Asthma is a chronic lung disease that has a significant economic impact, as well as an effect, on quality of life.
- The relationships of total and specific immunoglobulin (Ig) E to asthma are complex; however, studies show an association between IgE and the severity of asthma.
- Specific IgE, in particular, has a complex relationship with asthma because patients can be sensitized without a clinical reaction to the allergen.
- Total IgE elevations are seen in patients with atopic disease and pharmacotherapy can affect these levels.
- IgE as a biomarker provides a target for biologic therapy, which is critical for management of this disease.

INTRODUCTION

Asthma, a chronic inflammatory lung disorder marked with reversible airflow obstruction, is a multifactorial disease affected by both genetic and environmental factors. It is estimated to affect 7.8% of the United States population.[1] The annual economic burden of asthma in the United States is $56 billion. Overall, asthma mortality and health care utilization rates are decreasing; however, the societal and economic burden remains significant. It is classified as a public health concern, leading to approximately 14.4 million lost school days for children and 14.2 million lost work days for adults in 2008. Poorly controlled asthma has been shown to increase health care cost across a lifetime and to decrease productiveness.[2]

Phenotypes of asthma involve the idea of atopy, with the definition of atopy being a genetic susceptibility to produce immunoglobulin (Ig) E against nonpathogenic environmental allergens. IgE is the major immunoglobulin involved in an allergic response

Disclosure Statement: No disclosures.
[a] Allergy/Immunology, Children's Mercy Hospital, University of Missouri Kansas City School of Medicine, 2401 Gillham Road, Kansas City, MO 64108, USA; [b] Allergy/Immunology, University of Missouri Kansas City School of Medicine, 2411 Holmes Street, Kansas City, MO 64108, USA
* Corresponding author.
E-mail address: lrosenwasser334@gmail.com

Immunol Allergy Clin N Am 38 (2018) 587–597
https://doi.org/10.1016/j.iac.2018.06.007
0889-8561/18/© 2018 Elsevier Inc. All rights reserved.

immunology.theclinics.com

and parasitic infection.[3,4] A diagnosis of asthma and wheezing in childhood has been associated with elevated total IgE, and a high level of total IgE at 1 year of age predisposes a child to persistent wheezing and early sensitization to aeroallergens.[5] Inflammation in asthma can be triggered by both allergic and nonallergic mechanisms, which interact and result in the phenomenon of bronchoconstriction and bronchospasm.[6] The relationship of specific IgE and asthma is complicated because allergic sensitization can involve multiple allergens, which can have a different clinical effect on the patient.[7] Also, nonallergic factors, such as genetic makeup and environmental exposure, can influence the patient's symptoms. Sustained inflammation with continued IgE response, as in occupational exposure to an irritant, can also affect an asthmatic patient independent of allergic or atopic history.[7] All of these factors can affect how IgE is produced and interpreted, as well as its use as a marker for therapy in the individual patient.

Biologic therapies have improved outcomes of asthma. An aspect of therapy is identifying biomarkers that would characterize the disease and associate it with the most effective therapies. Biomarkers for all asthma phenotypes have not been identified. Multiple biomarkers have been studied in relation to disease progression and therapy, specifically blood eosinophils, exhaled nitric oxide, sputum eosinophils, and total and specific IgE.[8–10] The role of IgE as a biomarker is critical in understanding the progression of asthma, as well as in monitoring the effect of therapy.

PHENOTYPES OF ASTHMA

Identification of the phenotype of asthma is important to identify targets for innovative therapy, as well as for discovering methods for management and outcome prediction. Eosinophilic asthma and allergic asthma are the phenotypes most commonly associated with elevated IgE. Eosinophilic asthma is sometimes associated with nasal polyposis and peripheral eosinophilia, although the cutoff for eosinophilia is not well-defined and varies between clinical studies. Interleukin (IL)-5 recruits eosinophils and is pivotal in eosinophil differentiation, maturation, and survival. It has, therefore, emerged as a target for biotherapeutics. This phenotype of asthma has been shown to have a relationship to particular types of IgE but not necessarily total IgE levels in all aspects of this disease.[11] Allergic asthma, however, has a proven association with both total and specific IgE. Allergy and asthma are linked but only a subset of allergic patients develops asthma. An association between elevated total IgE and allergic asthma has been shown, and asthma prevalence was higher in children who have 2 parents with high total IgE.[11] Nonallergic asthma, in contrast to allergic asthma, has a lower family history association, which suggests more of an environmental role in its development. Nonallergic asthma can also be associated with elevated total IgE independent of atopy. There is a lack, however, of specific IgE, which is identified in allergic asthma.[7]

ASTHMA AND ALLERGEN INVOLVEMENT

There is a complex causal relationship between asthma and allergen sensitization. Allergens are environmental antigens that can induce specific IgE antibody production. Specific IgE is also known as allergen-specific IgE because it is specific for the allergens to which a patient is sensitized. IgE is a marker of atopy and, in epidemiologic studies, sensitization via positive skin test or IgE antibodies are a risk factor for asthma. This shows the interaction of total IgE, specific allergen IgE, and asthma because they create an atopic picture. Therefore, IgE mediates the reaction of allergens with asthma.[11] Allergens and asthma are linked; however, clinical symptoms produced as a result of sensitization rely on multiple factors.[5] Some of those factors include the dose of allergen, the route, and the patient's airway reactivity. For example, house dust mite IgE affects 25% to 30% of the world's population and is a major risk factor for asthma. In contrast, specific IgE to pollen is not a clear risk factor for asthma, although it is for allergic rhinitis.[7]

IMMUNOGLOBULIN E IN VIVO

Despite its low concentration and short half-life, IgE is biologically very active. It binds to high-affinity receptors on the surface of mast cells and produces a very specific and selective response to antigens. IgE-producing B cells have a long life, which results in a consistent allergic response over time. The IgE produced by allergic patients is specific for foreign antigens. The consistency of allergic response over time is related to this long lifespan of IgE-producing B cells and stability of mast cells in the skin. Allergens cross-link IgE bound to effector cells, such as mast cells and basophils, resulting in preformed mediator release and the production of new mediators that are responsible for both immediate and late responses.[11] This mediator release also involves eosinophil recruitment, although eosinophils can also be upregulated by effector T cells and group 2 innate lymphoid cells (ILC2s).[3,12]

Immunoglobulin E Synthesis

IgE-mediated immunoregulatory effects on dendritic cells drive a T helper cell type 2 (Th2) or type 2 inflammatory response that is a part of asthma characterization.[12] This inflammatory process is triggered on exposure to certain inhaled allergens that activate dendritic cells and airway epithelium, leading to the synthesis of specific IgE antibodies.[7] Synthesis of IgE can occur by the Th2-driven process of class switching, either by direct class switch recombination from IgM in germinal center B cells or potentially through sequential switch from IgM to IgG1, then from IgG1 to IgE; this can occur in B cells outside of germinal centers. Antigen presenting cells (APCs), such as dendritic cells, take up an inhaled allergen, process it, and present it via major histocompatibility class II to Th2 cells. This presentation leads to expression of IL-4 and IL-13. Signals provided by IL-4 or IL-13 activate transcription at the IgE isotype-specific switch region, leading to the process of class switching of B cells. A second signal is provided by the CD40 ligand, which activates DNA switch recombination. Class switching and, therefore, IgE synthesis generally occurs in the germinal center of lymphoid organs but also occurs in the respiratory and gastrointestinal mucosa of atopic patients.[7] Newly synthesized IgE can bind to basophils and mast cells via IgE receptors. After activation, these cells play a role in amplification of IgE production and Th2 cell differentiation.

Immunoglobulin E Receptors

There are 2 receptors for IgE, a low and a high-affinity receptor. The low-affinity receptor is FcεRII, expressed on the surface of B cells and hematopoietic cells, and the high-affinity receptor is FcεRI, which is expressed on mast cells, basophils, and APCs. The high-affinity receptor is expressed as a tetramer on mast cells and basophils, and as a trimer on APCs. Notably, respiratory viruses induce high-affinity receptor expression and signaling, which has a significant IgE response in turn.[3]

Laboratory Evaluation of Immunoglobulin E

Total and specific IgE are measured by immunoassay. Specific IgE can also be measured by skin prick and intradermal skin test methods; however, there is no quantitative number associated with it and there is a lack of full standardization. This, therefore, affects the value of clinical research associated with the testing. There are different versions of the immunoassays available, especially for specific IgE to aeroallergens that can trigger asthma. Total IgE is measured with a 2-site noncompetitive immunometric assay, through which anti-IgE antibody directed at the Fc region of IgE is fixed to a solid surface and captures IgE from the serum. After washing, a different anti-IgE antibody linked to an identifiable entity is added to detect captured IgE.[4] Specific IgE assays detect IgE that will bind to allergen fixed on a solid surface. There is a variability of levels of specific IgE detected by different techniques and reagents because the assay differs depending on which technique or reagent is used.

TYPE 2 IMMUNITY

With any discussion of asthma, the cells and cytokines that regulate the airway type 2 inflammation are a critical aspect. The type 2 immune response is characterized by production of interleukins, leading to critical responses to helminthic infections, as well as by a pathophysiological role in allergic diseases such as asthma. Th2 cells and ILC2s are the cells involved in airway inflammation and cytokines regulate this overall process.[12,13] Hence, controlling the type 2 inflammation of the lower airways would be a therapeutic target for control of asthma. IL-4 and IL-5 act in a sequential fashion to cause airway changes and IL-4 is important for primary sensitization.[13] IL-13 is theorized to be more important with secondary exposure to allergens.[13] Decreased expression of immunoregulatory cytokines, such as IL-12, IL-18, and interferon gamma, as well as increases in proinflammatory cytokines, such as tumor necrosis factor alpha, play a role in the inflammatory process.[13] Specific cytokines that work with the Th2 response are IL-4, IL-5, IL-9, and IL-13. Thymic stromal lymphoprotein (TSLP) is part of the IL-7 family and has increased expression via mast cells and airway epithelium in patients with asthma. It interacts with proinflammatory cytokines and recruits Th2 cells to the airway.[14] IL-25 and IL-33 are other cytokines that have a regulatory effect on airway inflammation. IL-33 is among the earliest signaling molecules to be released following epithelial damage. Its activation of Th2 cells results in promotion of the asthma phenotype.[15] Identifying cytokines is important to the recognition of targets for biologic therapy.

Type 2 ILC2s are a major part of this type 2 immunity. They are present in eosinophilic airway inflammation and have been identified in asthmatic patients. In addition to being key regulators and effectors in type 2 immune response, ILC2s have a role in tissue homeostasis and repair. They regulate eosinophils through production of IL-5 and response to helminthic parasites, as would be expected in a type 2 immune response.[16] ILC2s interact with both innate and adaptive immune systems, and dysregulation of this system leads to allergic manifestations such as asthma. Emerging research has shown that targeting the function of ILC2s can control the type 2 immune response. Subjects with allergic rhinosinusitis were noted to have elevated numbers of ILC2s in nasal polyps compared with controls, which was the first evidence that ILC2s have a role in allergic disease.[16] ILC2s induce Th2 responses by affecting T cells, which in turn leads to a B-cell effect. Because Th2 cells work with B cells to promote IgE production, they are central in allergic asthma and lung inflammation. With these noted effects, there is a pivotal role for ILC2 to drive an allergic response, which would indicate that modifying the ILC2 function can help prevent type 2 inflammation affecting the lung. Therefore, IgE is a marker of type 2 immune response and interference of this ILC2 response can affect IgE.[16] A study by Liu and colleagues[17] showed increased ILC2 in eosinophilic asthma subjects compared with controls of noneosinophilic asthmatics and subjects without asthma. Of note, there was also a statistically significant increase in levels of sputum eosinophils, exhaled nitric oxide, blood eosinophil counts, and IgE in the asthmatic subjects. This study's analysis did note that the biomarker best related to airway eosinophilic inflammation was ILC2, which was even more closely related than IgE. This introduces a new aspect into biomarker research because ILC2 had not previously been considered to have a large biomarker role.

ROLE OF IMMUNOGLOBULIN E

Specific IgE and total IgE are biomarkers for asthma of multiple phenotypes. Mechanisms regulating the production are still being studied. Specific IgE identifies sensitization to a suspected allergen. Increased total IgE levels are seen in patients with atopic diseases. The highest levels are seen in those with atopic dermatitis, followed by allergic asthma and allergic rhinitis.[4] Elevated total IgE can also be associated with parasitic infections, inflammatory disorders, hematologic disorders, and primary immunodeficiency disorders.[4] Both total and specific IgE levels are important from clinical and research perspectives because this can denote a certain asthma phenotype and provide a direction in management strategy.[10]

Specific Immunoglobulin E

Specific IgE is particularly useful in asthmatics for trigger avoidance with identification of certain allergens. High levels of specific IgE to allergen triggers are related to wheeze and decreased lung function.[18] These specific IgE levels mediate asthmatic responses in allergic individuals; however, the clinical expression of asthma is more complex because specific IgE denotes sensitization. Sensitization should be correlated to symptoms because an asymptomatic patient can have elevated levels of specific IgE that are irrelevant to the clinical picture.[19] Inflammatory and immunologic responses arising in bronchial mucosa following exposure to an allergen have been shown to modulate the developing reaction in an asthmatic subject.[18] Studies also show that elevated allergen-specific IgE levels are associated with more severe asthma.[18] Higher specific IgE levels can indicate more exposure and sensitization, which can result in worsened asthma. In particular, higher cockroach, dust mite, mouse, and cat-specific IgE levels are associated with poorer lung function.[18] Cat, dust mite, and mouse IgE are related to increased risk of exacerbation or hospitalization in asthmatics.[18] Again, levels must be correlated to symptoms that occur with exposure but, overall, the trend shows that severe asthmatics with high specific IgE are triggered by those particular allergens. In general, the presence of specific IgE to environmental allergens is more strongly associated with allergic asthma.

Total Immunoglobulin E

Total serum IgE levels are age-dependent, with atopic infants having earlier and steeper increases in their levels than nonatopic infants. Total IgE also varies by exogenic factors, including genetics, environment, and immune system status.[5] In particular, location should be taken into account when analyzing laboratory results owing to geographic variation in levels. In the absence of disease, IgE expression is tightly regulated. There is no transplacental transfer, as evidenced by low cord blood levels. The levels increase throughout childhood, with a peak in early puberty, and decrease throughout the adult years.[5] Total IgE levels are affected by multiple factors, including genetic, environmental, and immune system status. The pattern of IgE variation can differ significantly but, generally, total IgE levels greater than 333 IU/mL are strongly associated with atopy in children older than 14 years of age.[5] Corticosteroids can induce IgE production but decrease total IgE levels, especially in allergic bronchopulmonary aspergillosis (ABPA). IgE can be relatively resistant to steroid effects, therefore these changes can be less significant.[20] Other biomarkers, such as exhaled nitric oxide and sputum eosinophils, have been implicated in corticosteroid response in asthmatic subjects. These biomarkers did decrease with corticosteroid treatment; however, the significance of these findings is debatable and further study is needed.[20]

Increased total IgE can negatively correlate with lung function in patients with a history of asthma.[21] There is a noted relationship between IgE and eosinophils. High IgE concentrations can draw eosinophils to the site of an allergen patch test, and nonatopic controls who receive an atopic transfer of serum or intradermal purified antibody can also have noted eosinophil recruitment.[11] It has been theorized that total IgE changes in asthmatic patients are indirect measures of airway inflammation, as are eosinophils; however, this association is not fully studied. Thus, blocking IgE is a strategy to prevent or attenuate an allergic response.

Immunoglobulin E in Other Atopic Diseases

IgE has been identified in other atopic diseases and its role as a biomarker in these diseases continues to be studied. Elevated IgE has been noted in patients with atopic dermatitis; however, its specific role as a biomarker in this disease has not been clearly identified. In chronic urticaria, elevated IgE has been recognized as a potential biomarker based on studies showing an association between total IgE level and severity of the subject's chronic urticaria.[22] Regarding food allergy, specific IgE has been studied as a potential biomarker of clinical reactivity to the allergen. Baseline specific IgE in discussions of hen eggs and cow milk are important predictors of tolerance. With food allergy, however, component testing, such as with peanut, wheat, and eggs, has been identified as preferential for diagnostic marking.[23] Atopic disease does have a relationship to IgE, and elevated levels of IgE can be associated with disease severity and effect in certain cases.

BIOTHERAPEUTICS

Current targeted therapy in asthma includes anti-IgE therapy or anti–IL-5 agents. None of these biologic targeted treatments has been proven superior to others; however, their mechanisms of action are separate, although the end goal and result is improvement of severe asthma. As noted in **Table 1**, there are many biologic treatments that are currently available or under investigation.

Biologic therapy targeting IgE was the first biotherapy to be studied for use in asthma, with subsequent case reports demonstrating a benefit in ABPA.[28] Omalizumab is an anti-IgE monoclonal antibody used in asthmatics older than 12 years of age with uncontrolled severe persistent asthma. The range of recommended total IgE for omalizumab use is between 30 and 700 IU/mL; levels higher or lower than this range have an uncertain treatment benefit. High IgE levels greater than 1300 IU/mL can exclude patients from using omalizumab based on studies showing that the free IgE reduction in these cases is inconsequential, therefore resulting in minimal efficacy of treatment.[7] Also, important considerations before using omalizumab are the patient's weight and presence of a perennial allergen sensitization because certain weights and lack of a perennial allergen sensitization can exclude a patient from use of this drug.[29]

Omalizumab inhibits IgE interactions for receptors that are high and low affinity, and causes dissociation of high-affinity receptors from IgE. Omalizumab binds to the C3

Table 1 Biotherapeutics in asthma		
Drug	**Target**	**Effect**
Omalizumab (Xolair)	IgE	Decreases IgE with significant impact on severe persistent asthma
Quilizumab	IgE	Investigational; decreases IgE without significant impact on asthma
Ligelizumab	IgE	Investigational; greater decrease in IgE than omalizumab, and may be more effective in skin and inhalant response
Mepolizumab (Nucala)	IL-5	Improves eosinophilia in patients with moderate-to-severe eosinophilic asthma and improves control in these patients
Reslizumab (Cinqair)	IL-5	Improves eosinophilia in patients with moderate eosinophilic asthma and improves control in these patients
Benralizumab	IL-5Rα	Improves eosinophilia in patients with moderate-to-severe eosinophilic asthma and improves control in these patients
Dupilumab	IL-4Rα	Investigational in asthma (approved for atopic dermatitis); for uncontrolled persistent asthmatics, reduces exacerbations and increases forced expiratory volume in 1 second (FEV1)
Lebrikizumab	IL-13	Investigational; for uncontrolled asthmatics, no consistent significant change in exacerbations
Tralokinumab	IL-13	Investigational; for severe uncontrolled asthmatics, no significant reduction in exacerbations
REGN 3500	IL-33	Investigational with clinical trials currently underway in moderate asthmatics
AMG 157	TSLP	Investigational; reduces allergen-induced bronchoconstriction and inflammation in mild asthmatics

Data from Refs.[24–27]

region of the IgE Fc fragment, leading to complexes and, therefore, decreasing free IgE available to bind the IgE receptors.[30] Reduction in free IgE correlates with symptom control; however, the IgE levels do return to baseline after cessation of therapy.

The complex of omalizumab and IgE can interfere with detection via assay.[31] Due to continued accumulation of these complexes, as well as production of IgE, measured total IgE concentration can be increased by 3-fold to 5-fold because it reflects both free and omalizumab-bound IgE. Thus, in the setting of either asthma or ABPA, it is important to be aware of the assay being used and to use the same assay over a period of years because there is significant variability in the accuracy of different methods of total IgE measurement in the presence of omalizumab. Measurement of free IgE is difficult but methods have been developed. Studies have shown that free IgE levels can decrease by up to 95% with omalizumab treatment.[4] Based on the difficulties that can occur with measurement of IgE with omalizumab use, anti-IgE therapies that have rapid clearance from circulation without concern for interference in the assay are of interest for further study.

In ABPA, in which an IgE level of greater than 1000 ng/mL (or 416 IU/mL) is a major diagnostic criteria. IgE levels are often measured serially to assess response to therapy. In these patients, a decrease in total IgE of at least 35% correlates with improvement both clinically and radiographically. Given the formation of IgE-omalizumab complexes and their effect on total IgE levels, standard practice is not to follow total IgE levels following initiation of omalizumab in ABPA patients. A recent case report, however, suggests that total IgE levels will decrease in some ABPA patients despite the use of omalizumab and, therefore, total IgE levels could still be followed to evaluate treatment efficacy in select patients.[31]

Overall, omalizumab can reduce asthma exacerbations regardless of the initial IgE level and has shown to also be useful in the treatment of ABPA. IgE as a biomarker specifically for anti-IgE therapy is a complicated science, although it is based on a large amount of research on both disease processes and the relationship between IgE, the allergic disease process, and omalizumab.[7]

Antiinterleukin 5 Relationship

IL-5 is a key cytokine required for development, recruitment, and activation of eosinophils; therefore it plays a role in the phenotype of nonallergic hypereosinophilic asthma. It is an interleukin produced by Th2 cells, ILC2s, and mast cells. Inhibiting IL-5 reduces blood and sputum eosinophils and the current anti–IL-5 therapies on the market have been shown to have this effect. Mepolizumab and reslizumab, both monoclonal antibodies against IL-5, and benralizumab, a recently approved antibody against the IL-5 receptor alpha, have all been shown to reduce asthma exacerbations and peripheral eosinophilia in subjects with eosinophilic asthma.[32–35] A relationship has been noted between eosinophilic asthma and IgE, although the effect of anti–IL-5 therapy on IgE has not been clearly defined. Although eosinophilic asthma is a phenotype that is generally associated with nonallergic asthma, eosinophilia can also be present in allergic asthma. Therefore, patients with allergic asthma can also respond to anti–IL-5 therapy, in addition to anti-IgE therapy.

Blood and sputum eosinophilia have been noted in severe asthmatics in eosinophilic asthma, and sputum eosinophilia, in particular, correlates with higher total IgE. Sputum eosinophilia is less clearly associated with poorer control than peripheral eosinophilia. Enterotoxin-producing *Staphylococcus aureus* colonizes the upper airways of patients with eosinophilic asthma and IgE responses to this bacteria have been identified in this phenotype. A relationship was noted between the IgE produced to *Staphylococcus aureus* and severe asthma but this specific IgE can also be identified in the general population with asthma regardless of atopy history.[7] Because this IgE has been identified regardless of atopy, a relationship between eosinophilia and IgE can be made. IL-5 has a synergistic effect on the IL-4–induced production of IgE but, overall, it has more of a role in eosinophil production.[36] Therefore, a role for IgE in this phenotype of nonallergic asthma is supported.

Immunoglobulin E and Biotherapeutics Under Development

Biologic therapy remains an emerging science and many biologic agents remain under study. Therapies targeting additional cytokines and proinflammatory modulators such as TSLP are in development for therapy. AMG 157 is an anti-TSLP monoclonal antibody that attenuates early and late phase asthmatic responses in patients with allergen-induced reactions. In studies of subjects with mild allergic asthma, it was identified to reduce eosinophilia and exhaled nitric oxide.[37] This biologic therapy is groundbreaking because it is the first to target the underlying allergic inflammation by blocking the airway epithelium's response to the inhaled allergen. Epithelial cell involvement in asthma has also identified IL-25, IL-33, and interferon beta as potential targets for biotherapeutics.[37] Anti IL-13 drugs, such as lebrikizumab and tralokinumab, are also being investigated for use in patients with uncontrolled asthma, with variable results.[24] Although these biologics do not target IgE directly, they may still affect IgE levels indirectly.

Dupilumab is a monoclonal antibody to IL-4 receptor alpha, which is a component of both the IL-4 and IL-13 receptors. By blocking IL-4 and IL-13–mediated inflammation, dupilumab indirectly inhibits IgE production by preventing B cell IgE class switch. Dupilumab is approved for atopic dermatitis and in phase 3 trials for asthma. Dupilumab has been shown to reduce serum IgE levels, as well as other biomarkers such as exhaled nitric oxide.[32,38] Although it does not directly affect IgE function, it does decrease the production and, therefore, has a role in treatment of allergic asthma.[38]

Immunoglobulin E as a Biomarker for Response to Allergen Immunotherapy

Patients with asthma and identified specific IgE to environmental allergens can benefit from immunotherapy, which has been implicated in a reduction of total and specific IgE levels.[5] This has been evident specifically in house dust mite immunotherapy; however, all allergens used for immunotherapy had statistically significant reduction in total and specific IgE.[5] Immunotherapy has been postulated to alter production of mast cell mediators and specific IgE, which could affect patients with asthma. IL-4 decreased and IL-10 was induced in patients with asthma after immunotherapy, which leads to suppression of IgE production and amelioration of the triggered response to allergens seen in asthma patients[5,39]

SUMMARY

IgE use as a biomarker can be helpful in a multitude of ways, including diagnosis, treatment, and predicting the outcome of allergic disease. Regarding asthma, this identification is critical for early intervention and prevention of morbidity. As a part of an expanding list of biomarkers, IgE has an established role in defining phenotypes of asthma and its treatment. Elevated levels of specific IgE can be pathognomonic for allergic disease; identification of specific IgE is important for allergens that trigger asthma. Biotherapy targeting IgE has also been shown to improve outcomes in asthma; free IgE decreases significantly with omalizumab use. Overall, these findings suggest that IgE is a reliable biomarker and should be followed for certain phenotypes of asthma to ascertain improvement and appropriate therapeutic interventions.

REFERENCES

1. Centers for Disease Control and Prevention. Most recent asthma data. 2017. Available at: https://www.cdc.gov/asthma/most_recent_data.htm. Accessed January 11, 2018.
2. American Lung Association. Trends in asthma morbidity and mortality. [Web site] 2012. Available at: http://www.lung.org/assets/documents/research/asthma-trend-report.pdf. Accessed December 12, 2017.
3. Abbas AKL, Andrew H, Pillai S. Cellular and molecular immunology. 9th edition. Philadelphia: Elsevier; 2015.
4. Stone KD, Prussin C, Metcalfe DD. IgE, mast cells, basophils, and eosinophils. J Allergy Clin Immunol 2010;125(2 Suppl 2):S73–80.
5. Ahmad Al Obaidi AH, Mohamed Al Samarai AG, Yahya Al Samarai AK, et al. The predictive value of IgE as biomarker in asthma. J Asthma 2008;45(8):654–63.
6. Burrows B, Martinez FD, Halonen M, et al. Association of asthma with serum IgE levels and skin-test reactivity to allergens. N Engl J Med 1989;320(5):271–7.
7. Froidure A, Mouthuy J, Durham SR, et al. Asthma phenotypes and IgE responses. Eur Respir J 2016;47(1):304–19.
8. Warke TJ, Fitch PS, Brown V, et al. Exhaled nitric oxide correlates with airway eosinophils in childhood asthma. Thorax 2002;57(5):383–7.

9. Jatakanon A, Lim S, Kharitonov SA, et al. Correlation between exhaled nitric oxide, sputum eosinophils, and methacholine responsiveness in patients with mild asthma. Thorax 1998;53(2):91–5.

10. Szefler SJ, Wenzel S, Brown R, et al. Asthma outcomes: biomarkers. J Allergy Clin Immunol 2012;129(3 Suppl):S9–23.

11. Platts-Mills TA. The role of immunoglobulin E in allergy and asthma. Am J Respir Crit Care Med 2001;164(8 Pt 2):S1–5.

12. Djukanovic R, Hanania N, Busse W, et al. IgE-mediated asthma: new revelations and future insights. Respir Med 2016;112:128–9.

13. Kips JC. Cytokines in asthma. Eur Respir J Suppl 2001;34:24s–33s.

14. Barnes PJ. The cytokine network in asthma and chronic obstructive pulmonary disease. J Clin Invest 2008;118(11):3546–56.

15. Borish L, Steinke JW. Interleukin-33 in asthma: how big of a role does it play? Curr Allergy Asthma Rep 2011;11(1):7–11.

16. Bernink JH, Germar K, Spits H. The role of ILC2 in pathology of type 2 inflammatory diseases. Curr Opin Immunol 2014;31:115–20.

17. Liu T, Wu J, Zhao J, et al. Type 2 innate lymphoid cells: a novel biomarker of eosinophilic airway inflammation in patients with mild to moderate asthma. Respir Med 2015;109(11):1391–6.

18. Matsui EC, Sampson HA, Bahnson HT, et al. Allergen-specific IgE as a biomarker of exposure plus sensitization in inner-city adolescents with asthma. Allergy 2010; 65(11):1414–22.

19. Adkinson Jr, NFB, Bruce S, et al. Middleton's allergy principles and practice. 8th edition. 2014. p. 755.

20. Cowan DC, Taylor DR, Peterson LE, et al. Biomarker-based asthma phenotypes of corticosteroid response. J Allergy Clin Immunol 2015;135(4):877–83.e1.

21. Rajendra C, Zoratti E, Havstad S, et al. Relationships between total and allergen-specific serum IgE concentrations and lung function in young adults. Ann Allergy Asthma Immunol 2012;108(6):429–34.

22. Kessel A, Helou W, Bamberger E, et al. Elevated serum total IgE–a potential marker for severe chronic urticaria. Int Arch Allergy Immunol 2010;153(3):288–93.

23. Sato S, Yanagida N, Ohtani K, et al. A review of biomarkers for predicting clinical reactivity to foods with a focus on specific immunoglobulin E antibodies. Curr Opin Allergy Clin Immunol 2015;15(3):250–8.

24. Kim H, Ellis AK, Fischer D, et al. Asthma biomarkers in the age of biologics. Allergy Asthma Clin Immunol 2017;13:48.

25. Menzella F, Galeone C, Bertolini F, et al. Innovative treatments for severe refractory asthma: how to choose the right option for the right patient? J Asthma Allergy 2017;10:237–47.

26. Gauvreau GM, O'Byrne PM, Boulet LP, et al. Effects of an anti-TSLP antibody on allergen-induced asthmatic responses. N Engl J Med 2014;370(22):2102–10.

27. U.S. National Library of Medicine Clinical Trials. Study of safety, tolerability, and pharmacokinetics of multiple ascending doses of REGN3500 in adults with moderate asthma. 2017. Available at: https://clinicaltrials.gov/ct2/show/NCT02999711. Accessed January 15, 2018.

28. Voskamp A, Gillman A, Symons K, et al. Clinical efficacy and immunologic effects of omalizumab in allergic bronchopulmonary aspergillosis. J Allergy Clin Immunol Pract 2015;3(2):192–9.

29. Hilvering B, Pavord ID. What goes up must come down: biomarkers and novel biologicals in severe asthma. Clin Exp Allergy 2015;45(7):1162–9.

30. Pennington LF, Tarchevskaya S, Brigger D, et al. Structural basis of omalizumab therapy and omalizumab-mediated IgE exchange. Nat Commun 2016;7:11610.
31. Kelso JM. Following total IgE concentration in patients with allergic bronchopulmonary aspergillosis on omalizumab. J Allergy Clin Immunol Pract 2016;4(2): 364–5.
32. Patel TR, Sur S. IgE and eosinophils as therapeutic targets in asthma. Curr Opin Allergy Clin Immunol 2017;17(1):42–9.
33. Garcia G, Taillé C, Laveneziana P, et al. Anti-interleukin-5 therapy in severe asthma. Eur Respir Rev 2013;22(129):251–7.
34. Liu Y, Zhang S, Li DW, et al. Efficacy of anti-interleukin-5 therapy with mepolizumab in patients with asthma: a meta-analysis of randomized placebo-controlled trials. PLoS One 2013;8(3):e59872.
35. Castro M, Zangrilli J, Wechsler ME, et al. Reslizumab for inadequately controlled asthma with elevated blood eosinophil counts: results from two multicentre, parallel, double-blind, randomised, placebo-controlled, phase 3 trials. Lancet Respir Med 2015;3(5):355–66.
36. Pene J, Rousset F, Brière F, et al. Interleukin 5 enhances interleukin 4-induced IgE production by normal human B cells. The role of soluble CD23 antigen. Eur J Immunol 1988;18(6):929–35.
37. Darveaux J, Busse WW. Biologics in asthma–the next step toward personalized treatment. J Allergy Clin Immunol Pract 2015;3(2):152–60 [quiz: 161].
38. Wenzel S, Ford L, Pearlman D, et al. Dupilumab in persistent asthma with elevated eosinophil levels. N Engl J Med 2013;368(26):2455–66.
39. Bohm L, Maxeiner J, Meyer-Martin H, et al. IL-10 and regulatory T cells cooperate in allergen-specific immunotherapy to ameliorate allergic asthma. J Immunol 2015;194(3):887–97.

Urinary Leukotriene E_4 as a Biomarker of Exposure, Susceptibility, and Risk in Asthma: An Update

Bryce C. Hoffman, MD, Nathan Rabinovitch, MD, MPH*

KEYWORDS

- Urinary leukotriene E_4 • Montelukast • Cysteinyl leukotriene • Second-hand smoke
- Aspirin sensitivity • Headache • Sleep apnea

KEY POINTS

- Measurement of urinary LTE_4 ($uLTE_4$) can be a useful noninvasive method to assess changes in the rate of total body cysteinyl leukotriene (CysLT) levels.
- GPR99 is a unique high-affinity LTE_4 receptor that plays a role in respiratory mucus production.
- Genetic polymorphisms and obesity can alter CysLT production or receptor binding and are associated with increased asthma.
- $uLTE_4$ is a biomarker of exposure to atopic and nonatopic asthma triggers, recent asthma exacerbations, aspirin-exacerbated respiratory disease, and early development of childhood atopy.
- Increased $uLTE_4$ and the ratio of $uLTE_4$ to fractionated exhaled nitric oxide can be used to predict differential responses favoring initiation or step-up therapy with leukotriene receptor antagonists.

LEUKOTRIENE E_4 SYNTHESIS

Urinary leukotriene E_4 ($uLTE_4$) is a biomarker of total body cysteinyl leukotriene (CysLT) production and excretion. Leukotrienes are a family of lipid mediators derived from arachidonic acid through the 5-lipoxygenase pathway. They are produced by various

This article is an update of the previously published article on "Urinary leukotriene E_4 as a Biomarker of Exposure, Susceptibility, and Risk in Asthma" in the August 2012 issue of the *Immunology and Allergy Clinics of North America*.

Disclosure Statement: B.C. Hoffman and N. Rabinovitch declare no relationship with a commercial company that has a direct financial interest in subject matter or materials discussed in article or with a company making a competing product.

Department of Pediatrics, Division of Allergy and Immunology, National Jewish Health, 1400 Jackson Street, Denver, CO 80206, USA
* Corresponding author.
E-mail address: rabinovitchn@njhealth.org

leukocytes, hence the first part of their name (leuko). The triene part of the name refers to the number (3) of conjugated double bonds (alkenes). The first leukotriene to be synthesized, leukotriene A_4 (LTA_4), is formed through the conversion of arachidonic acid, located in membrane phospholipids, to 5-hydroperoxyeicosatetraenoic and LTA_4 through membrane-bound 5-lipoxygenase (5-LO) and 5-lipoxygenase-activating protein. The 5-LO inhibitor zileuton blocks this conversion step. In human mast cells, basophils, eosinophils, and macrophages, LTA_4 converts quickly either to LTB_4, mediated by leukotriene hydrolase, or to LTC_4 through the incorporation of glutathione (g-glutamyl-cysteinyl-glycine), mediated by LTC_4 synthase. LTC_4 is subsequently converted to LTD_4 and then to the stable end product LTE_4. Because of the incorporation of cysteine, LTC_4, LTD_4, and LTE_4 are called cysteinyl leukotrienes (**Fig. 1**).[1]

CYSTEINYL LEUKOTRIENE RECEPTORS

Both the cysteinyl leukotriene receptor 1 (CysLTR1) and cysteinyl leukotriene receptor 2 (CysLTR2) are constitutively expressed and upregulated in milieus with high cytokine levels.[2] CysLTR1 is expressed primarily on blood leukocytes such as monocytes/macrophages, eosinophils, basophils, mast cells, neutrophils, T and B lymphocytes, and on interstitial cells of the nasal mucosa and airway smooth muscle.[2,3] The cellular distribution of CysLTR1 suggests a positive feedback loop because many cells that express CysLT1R also synthesize CysLTs. Recent studies also suggest that activation of CysLTR2 may amplify responses to CysLTR1 in aspirin sensitive asthma.[4] Leukotriene receptor antagonists (LTRA) such as montelukast block CysLTR1 but not CysLTR2. CysLTR2 is highly expressed in heart tissue, coronary vessels, and different regions of the brain, with lower expression in peripheral blood cells.[5–7] Although unique functional characteristics of each receptor have not yet been clearly defined,[2] the differential distribution may indicate a greater role for CysLTs acting through CysLTR2 in cardiovascular diseases. Of the 3 CysLT isoforms (LTC_4, LTD_4, and LTE_4), LTE_4 has the weakest affinity for CysLTR1 and CysLTR2. As such, LTE_4 was thought of as a marker of CysLT formation and effect but not necessarily an important biological mediator in disease pathogenesis. Recently Bankova and colleagues[8] identified a high-affinity receptor for LTE_4 called GPR99, which is

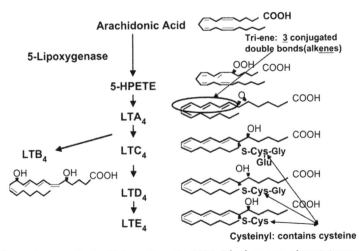

Fig. 1. The major steps in CysLT formation. 5-HPETE, 5-hydroperoxyeicosatetraenoic acid.

expressed on respiratory epithelial cells. This receptor seems to modulate mucin release and goblet cell numbers indicating a potential for direct therapeutic benefit of LTE$_4$ blockade in asthma. Another receptor related to LTE$_4$, the purinergic receptor P2Y12, is expressed on platelets and eosinophils and binds adenosine diphosphate without directly binding to LTE$_4$.[9] Nevertheless, a recent study showed that using clopidogrel to block P2Y12 in a mouse model of asthma decreased symptoms and cellular activation by LTE$_4$.[10]

MEASUREMENT OF URINARY LEUKOTRIENE E$_4$

Measurement of uLTE$_4$ can be a useful noninvasive method to assess changes in the rate of total body CysLT levels. Levels of LTE$_4$ are too low to measure in serum[11,12] but can be measured after excretion into the urine. Studies have shown that inhalation of LTC$_4$ or LTD$_4$ leads to a dose-dependent increase in uLTE$_4$.[13] Approximately 5% of airway CysLTs are eventually eliminated in the urine,[14] almost all in the form of uLTE$_4$, with little, if any, measurable urinary LTC$_4$ or LTD$_4$.[15] Measurements are often reported in picogram (pg) amounts per milligram (mg) of creatinine to control for urine dilution.

The primary methods of detection of uLTE$_4$ are mass spectrometry and enzyme-linked immunosorbent assay. Mass spectrometry has become the gold standard because it has been shown to have lower coefficients of variation and almost 100% recovery using spiked samples, indicating high sensitivity and precision.[16,17] Immunoassay absolute levels tend to be biased high compared with measurements after solid-phase extraction and reverse-phase high-performance liquid chromatography, indicating poor antibody specificity.[18,19] Therefore, immunoassays may overestimate uLTE$_4$ measurements. Enrichment procedures to further purify the urine have been devised that increase the specificity of the immunoassay[19] but these techniques are labor intensive and costly.

SOURCES OF URINARY LEUKOTRIENE E$_4$ VARIABILITY

Reported values for basal uLTE$_4$ levels in healthy individuals vary depending on the measurement technique and whether purification techniques are used in immunoassays. uLTE$_4$ levels seem to decrease with age, with one study reporting mean uLTE$_4$ values for healthy children of 50.7 pg/mg versus 36.7 pg/mg in healthy adults.[16] Obesity seems to increase leukotriene production, with a positive association demonstrated between uLTE$_4$ and waist to hip ratio.[20] Baek and colleagues[21] observed significant increases in uLTE$_4$ in obese asthmatic children after exercise challenge compared with normal-weight asthmatic children, suggesting that CysLTs may be contributing to the severity of symptoms in obese asthmatics.

Genetic polymorphisms within the leukotriene synthesis pathway or within the CysLT receptor genes are another source of individual variation resulting in variable production or uptake of CysLTs.[22] Wild-type expression of single-nucleotide polymorphisms in the LTC$_4$ synthase (LTC$_4$S-A444C) and CysLTR1 (CYSLTR1-T927C) genes were associated with increased uLTE$_4$ levels from baseline after asthma exacerbations.[23] The ALOX5 gene promoter region has a variable (3–7) number of tandem repeat sequences located in the Sp1-binding motif, 5 repeats being the wild-type. Carrying 2 non-5 tandem repeat sequences is associated with increased uLTE$_4$ levels, reduced lung function, and worse asthma control.[24] This polymorphism is more prevalent in African Americans,[24] suggesting that this population may be predisposed to increased leukotriene production. Because a variety of exposures may increase uLTE$_4$ levels (discussed later), gene interactions may differ depending on the type of environmental challenge and the pathway being studied.

URINARY LEUKOTRIENE E$_4$ AS A MARKER OF CYSTEINYL LEUKOTRIENE-MEDIATED DISEASES

Because many inflammatory mediators induce CysLT production, high uLTE$_4$ levels may indicate a heightened inflammatory state but do not necessarily suggest that CysLTs are important mediators of a particular disease or that treatment with leukotriene modifiers would be effective. Increased levels of uLTE$_4$ have been reported after episodes of unstable angina and acute myocardial infarction,[26] in coronary artery disease,[25] after coronary artery bypass surgery,[27] and in patients who have atopic dermatitis,[28] rheumatoid arthritis,[29] Crohn disease,[30] malignant astrocytoma,[31] and migraine headaches.[32] Some nonrandomized studies have reported efficacy of antileukotriene medications in the treatment of atopic dermatitis, with ongoing research into related agents.[33] Montelukast has also been reported to be effective in a regimen for new daily persistent headache.[34] This suggests potential off-target effects of the current LTRAs (CysLTR1 antagonists), because the brain and blood vessels contain predominantly CysLT2Rs as previously noted. There continues to be a lack of randomized studies showing that leukotriene-modifying medications are effective treatments for any of these diseases.

CYSTEINYL LEUKOTRIENES AND AIRWAY INFLAMMATION

The significance of CysLTs as key mediators and modulators in the pathogenesis of disease is better defined for asthma than for other diseases. Inhaled LTD$_4$ is a bronchoconstrictor that is 10,000 times more potent than histamine or methacholine.[35,36] In addition to their potent bronchoconstrictive properties, CysLTs induce other pathophysiologic responses characteristic of the inflammatory response in asthma. The first step in the allergic response, the movement of antibody-presenting dendritic cells from peripheral tissues to lymph nodes, is enhanced in the presence of CysLTs.[37] LTD$_4$ increases the proliferation of eosinophils and facilitates their recruitment into the airway by acting as a chemoattractant and boosting levels of adhesion molecules such as P-selectin.[38,39] In addition, CysLTs reduce eosinophil apoptosis and increase the production of mediators, such as interleukin 5, that increase eosinophil survival.[40,41] Group 2 innate lymphoid cells are another key cell type activated by CysLTs, in particular LTE$_4$, with evidence of enhanced chemotaxis, reduced apoptosis, and promotion of type 2 cytokine production.[42] Other noted effects of CysLTs include increased airway responsiveness to histamine and tissue edema secondary to vasodilation and increased microvascular permeability.[43,44] CysLTs may also play a role in structural changes in the airway that accompany chronic asthma, such as airway smooth muscle proliferation and remodeling.[45,46]

ASTHMA "TRIGGERS" AND URINARY LEUKOTRIENE E$_4$ LEVELS

Increased uLTE$_4$ levels are seen with a variety of asthma triggers. Levels are increased during early allergen-induced bronchoconstriction[47] and within 4 hours of exercise, returning to baseline within 24 hours,[48] and health effects that occur after these triggers are at least partially blocked by LTRAs.[48] uLTE$_4$ levels are also increased with exposure to particulate air pollution,[49] tobacco smoke exposure,[50] and upper respiratory infections. Piedimonte and colleagues[51] reported that uLTE$_4$ was 8-fold higher in infants who had bronchiolitis than in controls and was particularly increased in young infants who had an atopic/asthmatic background. Takahashi and colleagues[52] observed increased uLTE$_4$ levels in children infected with respiratory syncytial virus independently of atopic status. These associations support a clinical study that reported decreased virus-induced asthma exacerbations in children treated with LTRAs.[53]

URINARY LEUKOTRIENE E₄ AS A MARKER OF ASTHMA PREVALENCE AND SEVERITY

Some, but not all, studies have reported higher uLTE$_4$ levels in patients with asthma compared with nonasthmatics,[54–56] as well as increases related to asthma severity and lower lung function.[57,58] A study by Severien and colleagues[58] demonstrated associations between levels of uLTE$_4$ and intrathoracic gas volume, residual volume, forced expiratory volume in 1 second (FEV$_1$), and forced vital capacity. In addition, several studies have suggested that within-subject increases in uLTE$_4$ levels are associated with decreased asthma control.[59–62]

Multiple studies have shown associations between uLTE$_4$ levels and acute asthma exacerbations in pediatric[63] and adult[64] patients. Rabinovitch and colleagues also reported that uLTE$_4$ levels uniquely predicted risk for exacerbation in second-hand tobacco smoke (SHS)–related asthma, suggesting a distinct biological phenotype related to SHS exposure. This supposition is supported by randomized adult[65] and pediatric[62] studies that have reported greater sensitivity to LTRA therapy in patients exposed to secondary or primary tobacco smoke. Lang and colleagues[66] reported that children with indoor smoke exposure had worse asthma control, decreased FEV$_1$, and increased uLTE$_4$, with all smoke-exposed subjects suffering from increased respiratory infections.

URINARY LEUKOTRIENE E₄ AS A MARKER OF ASPIRIN-SENSITIVE ASTHMA

Increases in uLTE$_4$ have been consistently observed in individuals who have aspirin-exacerbated respiratory disease (AERD).[67–69] Smith and colleagues[67] reported that mean uLTE$_4$ levels at baseline measured 101 pg/mg in aspirin-sensitive asthmatic patients, 43 pg/mg in asthmatics who were not aspirin sensitive, and 34 pg/mg in healthy subjects. Other studies have shown that in asthmatic patients on inhaled corticosteroid (ICS) therapy, increased uLTE$_4$[70] and decreased CysLTR1[71] levels from baseline after aspirin challenge were diagnostic of patients with AERD. A recent study by Divekar and colleagues[72] described the utility of uLTE$_4$ to detect the presence of aspirin sensitivity in patients with asthma or chronic rhinosinusitis. They found that 89% of subjects with uLTE$_4$ level greater than 166 pg/mg had a history of aspirin sensitivity, and 92% of subjects having greater than 241 pg/mg had challenge-confirmed aspirin sensitivity.

URINARY LEUKOTRIENE E₄ AS A MARKER OF CHILDHOOD ATOPY

Recent studies have suggested that uLTE$_4$ might be a predictive marker for the development of atopy in preschool-age children. Marmarinos and colleagues[73] measured uLTE$_4$ by immunoassay in 96 preschool children with recurrent episodic wheeze and found significantly increased basal levels of uLTE$_4$ in atopic patients (507 pg/mg) versus nonatopics (283 pg/mg) and controls (271 pg/mg). Chiu and colleagues[74] studied a birth cohort of 182 children and found that elevated uLTE$_4$ ($\geq$500 pg/mg) was associated with elevated serum total IgE ($\geq$100 kU/L) at age 2 years and later on with the development of asthma at age 4 years.

URINARY LEUKOTRIENE E_4 AS A MARKER OF CHILDHOOD OBSTRUCTIVE SLEEP APNEA

High concentration of CysLTs and their receptors are found in adenotonsillar tissue particularly in children with obstructive sleep apnea (OSA).[75] Kaditis and colleagues[76] measured $uLTE_4$ in 19 children with OSA and found increased morning $uLTE_4$ levels in those with moderate-to-severe OSA (log 2.39 pg/mg) versus mild OSA (log 2.06 pg/mg) and controls (log 1.86 pg/mg). Predictors of obstructive apnea–hypopnea index in the study included CysLT concentration, tonsillar size, and body mass index. A subsequent study by Satdhabudha and colleagues[77] reported significantly decreased $uLTE_4$ in children with OSA after (708.6 pg/mg) than before (961.9 pg/mg) adenotonsillectomy, which was associated with improvements in the severity of OSA symptoms and quality of life.

URINARY LEUKOTRIENE E_4 AS A MARKER OF LEUKOTRIENE RECEPTOR ANTAGONISTS SUSCEPTIBILITY

Heterogeneity of responses to pharmacotherapy in asthma is of great practical interest. Clinical guidelines recommend that steroid-naive children with mild to moderate persistent asthma should be started on STEP-2 therapy with a low-dose ICS therapy such as low-dose fluticasone propionate (FP). Alternative choices for STEP-2 therapy include an LTRA such as montelukast. In two different publications based on the same randomized crossover study, Szefler and colleagues[78] and Zeiger and colleagues[79] reported significant individual variability in response to STEP-2 therapy with low-dose FP or montelukast.

Elevated FeNO levels were associated with significant FEV_1 and asthma control day (ACD) responses to FP and to a better FP than montelukast response. In contrast, $uLTE_4$ levels greater than 100 pg/mg (measured with immunoassay in purified urine) were 3.2 times as likely to show a significant ($\geq7.5\%$) FEV_1 response to montelukast therapy compared to children with lower levels. Cai and colleagues[80] studied lung function responses to montelukast in 61 patients who had asthma and concluded that patients with $uLTE_4$ levels greater than 200 pg/mg (measured by immunoassay in unpurified urine) were 3.5 times more likely to respond to LTRAs compared to those with lower levels.

Rabinovitch and colleagues[62] reported that $uLTE_4$-related albuterol usage and response to montelukast was related to the ratio of $uLTE_4$ to FeNO ($uLTE_4$/FeNO). A subsequent post hoc analysis of the Szefler and colleagues'[78] study data as well as data from a second National Institutes of Health–sponsored randomized pediatric asthma controller trial reported that $uLTE_4$ levels were associated with responses to either low-dose FP or montelukast therapy, whereas $uLTE_4$/FeNO levels were associated with a better FEV_1 and ACD response to montelukast compared with FP therapy.[81] Of the children with a better ($\geq5\%$) FEV_1 response to montelukast than FP therapy, 86% had $uLTE_4$/FeNO ratios of 4 or above, suggesting that children with low $uLTE_4$/FeNO ratios are highly unlikely to respond preferentially to montelukast monotherapy. These biomarker patterns might suggest a model of biological heterogeneity related to STEP-2 medications (**Fig. 2**). In this model, high FeNO levels, indicating allergic airway inflammation, are associated with a clinically significant response to ICS therapy and a better response to ICS than to LTRA therapy. In contrast, high $uLTE_4$ levels, indicating both allergic and nonallergic airway inflammation (as with cigarette smoke or ambient air pollution exposure), are associated with clinically significant responses to both ICS and LTRA therapy. As such, a high ratio of $uLTE_4$/FeNO, indicating predominantly nonallergic airway inflammation largely

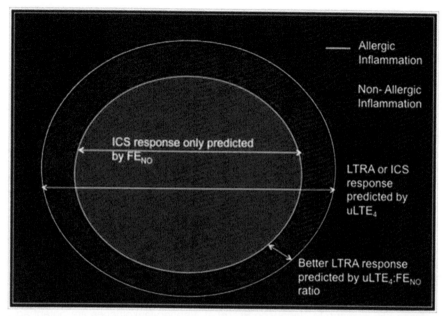

Fig. 2. Model of biomarker associations with STEP-2 therapy and related biological phenotypes. High FeNO levels, indicating allergic airway inflammation, are associated with a clinically significant response to low-dose ICS therapy and a better ICS than LTRA response. In contrast, high uLTE$_4$ levels, indicating both allergic and nonallergic airway inflammation (as with cigarette smoke or ambient air pollution exposure), are associated with clinically significant responses to both ICS and LTRA therapy. High uLTE$_4$/FeNO ratios, indicating predominantly nonallergic airway inflammation largely resistant to ICS therapy, are associated with a better response to LTRA than to ICS therapy.

resistant to ICS therapy, may be associated with a better response to LTRA than to ICS therapy.

Children with uncontrolled asthma despite the use of low-dose ICS should be started on STEP-3 therapy, which can be an increase in ICS dose to a medium-dose ICS, addition of a long-acting beta agonist (LABA), or addition of an LTRA. Rabinovitch and colleagues[82] reported that increased levels of uLTE$_4$ demonstrated a nonsignificant trend ($P = .053$) to an FEV$_1$ response favoring LTRA over LABA step-up therapy. A differential response comparing ICS with LTRA step-up was not apparent. Each doubling of the uLTE$_4$ level at baseline was associated with a 3.3% increase in FEV$_1$ response to LTRA step-up and a 2.2% increase with ICS step-up.

Predicting susceptibility to LTRA therapy has also been studied in OSA. Sunkonkit and colleagues[83] found an association between uLTE$_4$ and response to montelukast in children with mild OSA, with a mean uLTE$_4$ of 2952 pg/mg in responders versus 978 pg/mg in nonresponders (measured by immunoassay). Further studies are needed to assess the application of uLTE$_4$ as a marker for LTRA susceptibility in other diseases.

SUMMARY

Measurement of uLTE$_4$ is a sensitive and noninvasive method of assaying total body CysLT production and changes in CysLT production. Recent studies have reported on novel LTE$_4$ receptor interactions and genetic polymorphisms causing CysLT variability. The applications of uLTE$_4$ as a biomarker continue to expand, including evaluation of environmental exposures, asthma severity risk, aspirin sensitivity, predicting atopy in preschool age children, obstructive sleep apnea, and predicting susceptibility to leukotriene receptor antagonists.

REFERENCES

1. Busse W, Kraft M. Cysteinyl leukotrienes in allergic inflammation: strategic target for therapy. Chest 2005;127(4):1312–26.
2. Woszczek G, Chen LY, Nagineni S, et al. IFN-gamma induces cysteinyl leukotriene receptor 2 expression and enhances the responsiveness of human endothelial cells to cysteinyl leukotrienes. J Immunol 2007;178(8):5262–70.
3. Figueroa DJ, Breyer RM, Defoe SK, et al. Expression of the cysteinyl leukotriene 1 receptor in normal human lung and peripheral blood leukocytes. Am J Respir Crit Care Med 2001;163(1):226–33.
4. Liu T, Barrett NA, Kanaoka Y, et al. Type 2 cysteinyl leukotriene receptors drive IL-33-dependent type 2 immunopathology and aspirin sensitivity. J Immunol 2018;200(3):915–27.
5. Pedersen KE, Bochner BS, Undem BJ. Cysteinyl leukotrienes induce P-selectin expression in human endothelial cells via a non-CysLT1 receptor-mediated mechanism. J Pharmacol Exp Ther 1997;281(2):655–62.
6. Datta YH, Romano M, Jacobson BC, et al. Peptido-leukotrienes are potent agonists of von Willebrand factor secretion and P-selectin surface expression in human umbilical vein endothelial cells. Circulation 1995;92(11):3304–11.
7. Hui Y, Cheng Y, Smalera I, et al. Directed vascular expression of human cysteinyl leukotriene 2 receptor modulates endothelial permeability and systemic blood pressure. Circulation 2004;110(21):3360–6.
8. Bankova LG, Lai J, Yoshimoto E, et al. Leukotriene E4 elicits respiratory epithelial cell mucin release through the G-protein-coupled receptor, GPR99. Proc Natl Acad Sci U S A 2016;113(22):6242–7.
9. Paruchuri S, Tashimo H, Feng C, et al. Leukotriene E4-induced pulmonary inflammation is mediated by the P2Y12 receptor. J Exp Med 2009;206(11):2543–55.
10. Suh DH, Trinh HK, Liu JN, et al. P2Y12 antagonist attenuates eosinophilic inflammation and airway hyperresponsiveness in a mouse model of asthma. J Cell Mol Med 2016;20(2):333–41.
11. Volovitz B, Nathanson I, DeCastro G, et al. Relationship between leukotriene C4 and an uteroglobin-like protein in nasal and tracheobronchial mucosa of children. Implication in acute respiratory illnesses. Int Arch Allergy Appl Immunol 1988; 86(4):420–5.
12. Heavey DJ, Soberman RJ, Lewis RA, et al. Critical considerations in the development of an assay for sulfidopeptide leukotrienes in plasma. Prostaglandins 1987; 33(5):693–708.
13. Tagari P, Rasmussen JB, Delorme D, et al. Comparison of urinary leukotriene E4 and 16-carboxytetranordihydro leukotriene E4 excretion in allergic asthmatics after inhaled antigen. Eicosanoids 1990;3(2):75–80.
14. Kumlin M, Dahlén B, Björck T, et al. Urinary excretion of leukotriene E4 and 11-dehydro-thromboxane B2 in response to bronchial provocations with allergen, aspirin, leukotriene D4, and histamine in asthmatics. Am Rev Respir Dis 1992; 146(1):96–103.
15. Huber M, Müller J, Leier I, et al. Metabolism of cysteinyl leukotrienes in monkey and man. Eur J Biochem 1990;194(1):309–15.

16. Armstrong M, Liu AH, Harbeck R, et al. Leukotriene-E4 in human urine: comparison of on-line purification and liquid chromatography-tandem mass spectrometry to affinity purification followed by enzyme immunoassay. J Chromatogr B Analyt Technol Biomed Life Sci 2009;877(27):3169–74.

17. Kishi N, Mano N, Asakawa N. Direct injection method for quantitation of endogenous leukotriene E4 in human urine by liquid chromatography/electrospray ionization tandem mass spectrometry with a column-switching technique. Anal Sci 2001;17(6):709–13.

18. Kumlin M. Measurement of leukotrienes in humans. Am J Respir Crit Care Med 2000;161(2 Pt 2):S102–6.

19. Westcott JY, Maxey KM, MacDonald J, et al. Immunoaffinity resin for purification of urinary leukotriene E4. Prostaglandins Other Lipid Mediat 1998;55(5–6): 301–21.

20. Bäck M, Avignon A, Stanke-Labesque F, et al. Leukotriene production is increased in abdominal obesity. PLoS One 2014;9(12):e104593.

21. Baek HS, Choi JH, Oh JW, et al. Leptin and urinary leukotriene E4 and 9α,11β-prostaglandin F2 release after exercise challenge. Ann Allergy Asthma Immunol 2013;111(2):112–7.

22. Kalayci O, Birben E, Sackesen C, et al. ALOX5 promoter genotype, asthma severity and LTC production by eosinophils. Allergy 2006;61(1):97–103.

23. Bizzintino JA, Khoo SK, Zhang G, et al. Leukotriene pathway polymorphisms are associated with altered cysteinyl leukotriene production in children with acute asthma. Prostaglandins Leukot Essent Fatty Acids 2009;81(1):9–15.

24. Mougey E, Lang JE, Allayee H, et al. ALOX5 polymorphism associates with increased leukotriene production and reduced lung function and asthma control in children with poorly controlled asthma. Clin Exp Allergy 2013;43(5):512–20.

25. Hakonarson H, Thorvaldsson S, Helgadottir A, et al. Effects of a 5-lipoxygenase-activating protein inhibitor on biomarkers associated with risk of myocardial infarction: a randomized trial. JAMA 2005;293(18):2245–56.

26. Carry M, Korley V, Willerson JT, et al. Increased urinary leukotriene excretion in patients with cardiac ischemia. In vivo evidence for 5-lipoxygenase activation. Circulation 1992;85(1):230–6.

27. Allen SP, Sampson AP, Piper PJ, et al. Enhanced excretion of urinary leukotriene E4 in coronary artery disease and after coronary artery bypass surgery. Coron Artery Dis 1993;4(10):899–904.

28. Hishinuma T, Suzuki N, Aiba S, et al. Increased urinary leukotriene E4 excretion in patients with atopic dermatitis. Br J Dermatol 2001;144(1):19–23.

29. Nakamura H, Hishinuma T, Suzuki N, et al. Difference in urinary 11-dehydro TXB2 and LTE4 excretion in patients with rheumatoid arthritis. Prostaglandins Leukot Essent Fatty Acids 2001;65(5–6):301–6.

30. Kim JH, Tagari P, Griffiths AM, et al. Levels of peptidoleukotriene E4 are elevated in active Crohn's disease. J Pediatr Gastroenterol Nutr 1995;20(4):403–7.

31. Simmet T, Luck W, Winking M, et al. Identification and characterization of cysteinyl-leukotriene formation in tissue slices from human intracranial tumors: evidence for their biosynthesis under in vivo conditions. J Neurochem 1990; 54(6):2091–9.

32. Ince H, Aydin Ö, Alaçam H, et al. Urinary leukotriene E4 and prostaglandin F2a concentrations in children with migraine: a randomized study. Acta Neurol Scand 2014;130(3):188–92.

33. Yanes DA, Mosser-Goldfarb JL. Emerging therapies for atopic dermatitis: the prostaglandin/leukotriene pathway. J Am Acad Dermatol 2018;78(3S1):S71–5.

34. Nierenburg H, Newman LC. Update on new daily persistent headache. Curr Treat Options Neurol 2016;18(6):25.
35. Sjöström M, Johansson AS, Schröder O, et al. Dominant expression of the CysLT2 receptor accounts for calcium signaling by cysteinyl leukotrienes in human umbilical vein endothelial cells. Arterioscler Thromb Vasc Biol 2003;23(8): e37–41.
36. Gyllfors P, Kumlin M, Dahlén SE, et al. Relation between bronchial responsiveness to inhaled leukotriene D4 and markers of leukotriene biosynthesis. Thorax 2005;60(11):902–8.
37. Robbiani DF, Finch RA, Jäger D, et al. The leukotriene C(4) transporter MRP1 regulates CCL19 (MIP-3beta, ELC)-dependent mobilization of dendritic cells to lymph nodes. Cell 2000;103(5):757–68.
38. Kanwar S, Johnston B, Kubes P. Leukotriene C4/D4 induces P-selectin and sialyl Lewis(x)-dependent alterations in leukocyte kinetics in vivo. Circ Res 1995;77(5): 879–87.
39. Lee E, Robertson T, Smith J, et al. Leukotriene receptor antagonists and synthesis inhibitors reverse survival in eosinophils of asthmatic individuals. Am J Respir Crit Care Med 2000;161(6):1881–6.
40. Mellor EA, Austen KF, Boyce JA. Cysteinyl leukotrienes and uridine diphosphate induce cytokine generation by human mast cells through an interleukin 4-regulated pathway that is inhibited by leukotriene receptor antagonists. J Exp Med 2002;195(5):583–92.
41. Laitinen A, Lindqvist A, Halme M, et al. Leukotriene E(4)-induced persistent eosinophilia and airway obstruction are reversed by zafirlukast in patients with asthma. J Allergy Clin Immunol 2005;115(2):259–65.
42. Salimi M, Stöger L, Liu W, et al. Cysteinyl leukotriene E4 activates human group 2 innate lymphoid cells and enhances the effect of prostaglandin D2 and epithelial cytokines. J Allergy Clin Immunol 2017;140(4):1090–100.e1.
43. Bisgaard H, Olsson P, Bende M. Effect of leukotriene D4 on nasal mucosal blood flow, nasal airway resistance and nasal secretion in humans. Clin Allergy 1986; 16(4):289–97.
44. Hay DW, Torphy TJ, Undem BJ. Cysteinyl leukotrienes in asthma: old mediators up to new tricks. Trends Pharmacol Sci 1995;16(9):304–9.
45. Henderson WR, Chiang GK, Tien YT, et al. Reversal of allergen-induced airway remodeling by CysLT1 receptor blockade. Am J Respir Crit Care Med 2006; 173(7):718–28.
46. Espinosa K, Bossé Y, Stankova J, et al. CysLT1 receptor upregulation by TGF-beta and IL-13 is associated with bronchial smooth muscle cell proliferation in response to LTD4. J Allergy Clin Immunol 2003;111(5):1032–40.
47. Smith CM, Christie PE, Hawksworth RJ, et al. Urinary leukotriene E4 levels after allergen and exercise challenge in bronchial asthma. Am Rev Respir Dis 1991; 144(6):1411–3.
48. Hallstrand TS, Moody MW, Wurfel MM, et al. Inflammatory basis of exercise-induced bronchoconstriction. Am J Respir Crit Care Med 2005;172(6):679–86.
49. Rabinovitch N, Silveira L, Gelfand EW, et al. The response of children with asthma to ambient particulate is modified by tobacco smoke exposure. Am J Respir Crit Care Med 2011;184(12):1350–7.
50. Rabinovitch N, Strand M, Gelfand EW. Particulate levels are associated with early asthma worsening in children with persistent disease. Am J Respir Crit Care Med 2006;173(10):1098–105.

51. Piedimonte G, Renzetti G, Auais A, et al. Leukotriene synthesis during respiratory syncytial virus bronchiolitis: influence of age and atopy. Pediatr Pulmonol 2005; 40(4):285–91.

52. Takahashi Y, Ichikawa M, Nawate M, et al. Clinical evaluation of urinary leukotriene e4 levels in children with respiratory syncytial virus infection. Arerugi 2003;52(12):1132–7 [in Japanese].

53. Bisgaard H, Zielen S, Garcia-Garcia ML, et al. Montelukast reduces asthma exacerbations in 2- to 5-year-old children with intermittent asthma. Am J Respir Crit Care Med 2005;171(4):315–22.

54. Asano K, Lilly CM, O'Donnell WJ, et al. Diurnal variation of urinary leukotriene E4 and histamine excretion rates in normal subjects and patients with mild-to-moderate asthma. J Allergy Clin Immunol 1995;96(5 Pt 1):643–51.

55. Yamamoto H, Kuramitsu K, Houya I, et al. Clinical evaluation of urinary leukotriene E4 levels in asymptomatic bronchial asthma. Arerugi 1996;45(10):1106–11 [in Japanese].

56. Suzuki N, Hishinuma T, Abe F, et al. Difference in urinary LTE4 and 11-dehydro-TXB2 excretion in asthmatic patients. Prostaglandins Other Lipid Mediat 2000; 62(4):395–403.

57. Vachier I, Kumlin M, Dahlén SE, et al. High levels of urinary leukotriene E4 excretion in steroid treated patients with severe asthma. Respir Med 2003;97(11): 1225–9.

58. Severien C, Artlich A, Jonas S, et al. Urinary excretion of leukotriene E4 and eosinophil protein X in children with atopic asthma. Eur Respir J 2000;16(4): 588–92.

59. Kurokawa K, Tanaka H, Tanaka S, et al. Circadian characteristics of urinary leukotriene E(4) in healthy subjects and nocturnal asthmatic patients. Chest 2001; 120(6):1822–8.

60. Bellia V, Bonanno A, Cibella F, et al. Urinary leukotriene E4 in the assessment of nocturnal asthma. J Allergy Clin Immunol 1996;97(3):735–41.

61. Rabinovitch N, Zhang L, Gelfand EW. Urine leukotriene E4 levels are associated with decreased pulmonary function in children with persistent airway obstruction. J Allergy Clin Immunol 2006;118(3):635–40.

62. Rabinovitch N, Strand M, Stuhlman K, et al. Exposure to tobacco smoke increases leukotriene E4-related albuterol usage and response to montelukast. J Allergy Clin Immunol 2008;121(6):1365–71.

63. Rabinovitch N, Reisdorph N, Silveira L, et al. Urinary leukotriene E$_4$ levels identify children with tobacco smoke exposure at risk for asthma exacerbation. J Allergy Clin Immunol 2011;128(2):323–7.

64. Green SA, Malice MP, Tanaka W, et al. Increase in urinary leukotriene LTE4 levels in acute asthma: correlation with airflow limitation. Thorax 2004;59(2):100–4.

65. Lazarus SC, Chinchilli VM, Rollings NJ, et al. Smoking affects response to inhaled corticosteroids or leukotriene receptor antagonists in asthma. Am J Respir Crit Care Med 2007;175(8):783–90.

66. Lang JE, Dozor AJ, Holbrook JT, et al. Biologic mechanisms of environmental tobacco smoke in children with poorly controlled asthma: results from a multicenter clinical trial. J Allergy Clin Immunol Pract 2013;1(2):172–80.

67. Smith CM, Hawksworth RJ, Thien FC, et al. Urinary leukotriene E4 in bronchial asthma. Eur Respir J 1992;5(6):693–9.

68. Christie PE, Tagari P, Ford-Hutchinson AW, et al. Urinary leukotriene E4 concentrations increase after aspirin challenge in aspirin-sensitive asthmatic subjects. Am Rev Respir Dis 1991;143(5 Pt 1):1025–9.

69. Oosaki R, Mizushima Y, Mita H, et al. Urinary leukotriene E4 and 11-dehydro-thromboxane B2 in patients with aspirin-sensitive asthma. Allergy 1997;52(4): 470–3.

70. Sanak M, Kiełbasa B, Bochenek G, et al. Exhaled eicosanoids following oral aspirin challenge in asthmatic patients. Clin Exp Allergy 2004;34(12):1899–904.

71. Sousa AR, Parikh A, Scadding G, et al. Leukotriene-receptor expression on nasal mucosal inflammatory cells in aspirin-sensitive rhinosinusitis. N Engl J Med 2002; 347(19):1493–9.

72. Divekar R, Hagan J, Rank M, et al. Diagnostic Utility of Urinary LTE4 in Asthma, Allergic Rhinitis, Chronic Rhinosinusitis, Nasal Polyps, and Aspirin Sensitivity. J Allergy Clin Immunol Pract 2016;4(4):665–70.

73. Marmarinos A, Saxoni-Papageorgiou P, Cassimos D, et al. Urinary leukotriene E4 levels in atopic and non-atopic preschool children with recurrent episodic (viral) wheezing: a potential marker? J Asthma 2015;52(6):554–9.

74. Chiu CY, Tsai MH, Yao TC, et al. Urinary LTE4 levels as a diagnostic marker for IgE-mediated asthma in preschool children: a birth cohort study. PLoS One 2014;9(12):e115216.

75. Tsaoussoglou M, Lianou L, Maragozidis P, et al. Cysteinyl leukotriene receptors in tonsillar B- and T-lymphocytes from children with obstructive sleep apnea. Sleep Med 2012;13(7):879–85.

76. Kaditis AG, Alexopoulos E, Chaidas K, et al. Urine concentrations of cysteinyl leukotrienes in children with obstructive sleep-disordered breathing. Chest 2009; 135(6):1496–501.

77. Satdhabudha A, Sritipsukho P, Manochantr S, et al. Urine cysteinyl leukotriene levels in children with sleep disordered breathing before and after adenotonsillectomy. Int J Pediatr Otorhinolaryngol 2017;94:112–6.

78. Szefler SJ, Phillips BR, Martinez FD, et al. Characterization of within-subject responses to fluticasone and montelukast in childhood asthma. J Allergy Clin Immunol 2005;115(2):233–42.

79. Zeiger RS, Szefler SJ, Phillips BR, et al. Response profiles to fluticasone and montelukast in mild-to-moderate persistent childhood asthma. J Allergy Clin Immunol 2006;117(1):45–52.

80. Cai C, Yang J, Hu S, et al. Relationship between urinary cysteinyl leukotriene E4 levels and clinical response to antileukotriene treatment in patients with asthma. Lung 2007;185(2):105–12.

81. Rabinovitch N, Graber NJ, Chinchilli VM, et al. Urinary leukotriene E4/exhaled nitric oxide ratio and montelukast response in childhood asthma. J Allergy Clin Immunol 2010;126(3):545–51.e1-4.

82. Rabinovitch N, Mauger DT, Reisdorph N, et al. Predictors of asthma control and lung function responsiveness to step 3 therapy in children with uncontrolled asthma. J Allergy Clin Immunol 2014;133(2):350–6.

83. Sunkonkit K, Sritippayawan S, Veeravikrom M, et al. Urinary cysteinyl leukotriene E4 level and therapeutic response to montelukast in children with mild obstructive sleep apnea. Asian Pac J Allergy Immunol 2017;35(4):233–8.

Periostin and Dipeptidyl Peptidase-4

Potential Biomarkers of Interleukin 13 Pathway Activation in Asthma and Allergy

Claire Emson, PhD*, Tuyet-Hang Pham, MS, Scott Manetz, PhD,
Paul Newbold, PhD

KEYWORDS

- Asthma • Allergy • Biomarker • DPP-4 • IL-13 • Periostin

KEY POINTS

- Periostin and dipeptidyl peptidase-4 (DPP-4) are both induced by interleukin (IL)-13 and can be measured in serum, making them potential biomarkers to guide anti–IL-13–directed therapy.
- Both proteins show increased expression in asthma and other diseases with type 2 inflammation, including atopic dermatitis (AD) and chronic rhinosinusitis with nasal polyps.
- Both proteins also have confounders to their expression, including age, induction by profibrotic factors, body mass index (BMI), association with malignancies, and use of corticosteroids, which may have an impact on their specificity for type 2–driven disease.
- They demonstrate differences in their relationship with other type 2 biomarkers and no correlation with each other in serum, indicating they may be related to different aspects of IL-13–directed biology.
- Both have been used in clinical trials with anti–IL-13 monoclonal antibodies in severe asthma demonstrating enhanced efficacy in biomarker high subgroups; DPP-4 has also shown similar potential in a clinical trial in AD indicating their potential as biomarkers of IL-13–driven diseases.

INTRODUCTION

IL-13 has been identified as a potential central effector cytokine in asthma and may contribute to many key pathologic features, including airway hyper-responsiveness, mucus production, airway remodeling, and structural changes, promoting B-cell proliferation and inducing class switching to immunoglobulin (Ig)G4 and IgE as well as promoting eosinophil survival, activation, and recruitment.[1] Although production of

Disclosures: All authors are employees of MedImmune except P. Newbold who is associated with AstraZeneca.
MedImmune, One MedImmune Way, Gaithersburg, MD 20878, USA
* Corresponding author. One MedImmune Way, Gaithersburg, MD 20878.
E-mail address: emsonC@medimmune.com

Immunol Allergy Clin N Am 38 (2018) 611–628
https://doi.org/10.1016/j.iac.2018.06.004
0889-8561/18/© 2018 Elsevier Inc. All rights reserved.
immunology.theclinics.com

IL-13 can be inhibited by inhaled corticosteroids (ICS), there is a proportion of uncontrolled asthma patients who, despite treatment with high-dosage ICS and systemic corticosteroids, have elevated levels of IL-13 in sputum.[2]

Hence, the IL-13 pathway has been identified as a potential therapeutic target in severe asthma and allergic disease with selective monoclonal antibody therapies. Because there is heterogeneity of molecular mechanisms in asthma, it was hypothesized that to identify asthma patients with evidence of IL-13 pathway activation, a biomarker to direct anti–IL-13 therapy may be necessary.

Although it is possible to measure IL-13 levels in sputum, sputum induction and processing is a specialized technique and is not feasible in most clinical practice situations. Therefore, a blood-based sampling system is preferable. IL-13 concentrations in serum and plasma are generally below the level of reliable detection of most IL-13 assays (although more sensitive methods have been reported[3]); therefore, a surrogate of IL-13 pathway activation in the airway that is measurable in blood is required. This review evaluates the potential of 2 candidates of IL-13 pathway activation—serum periostin and dipeptidyl peptidase-4 (DPP-4)—for identifying asthma and allergic patients who may gain benefit from anti–IL-13–directed therapy (**Fig. 1**).

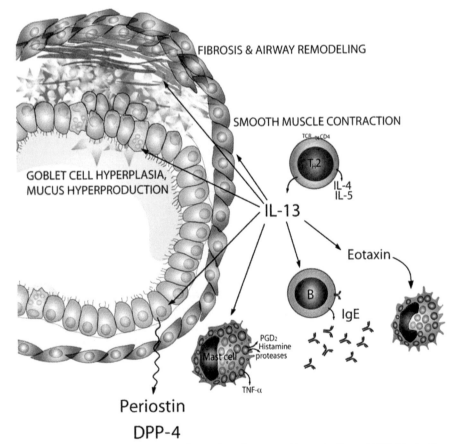

Fig. 1. IL-13 and its role in the pathology of T2 disease and in periostin and DPP-4 induction. (*Modified from* Brightling CE, She D, Ranade K, et al. Efficacy and safety of tralokinumab, an anti-IL-13 monoclonal antibody, in a phase 2b study of uncontrolled severe asthma. Am J Respir Crit Care Med 2014;189:A6670; with permission.)

BIOLOGY IN ASTHMA AND ALLERGY
Periostin

Background

Periostin (encoded by the gene POSTN) is a 92-kDa–secreted N-glycoprotein protein of the fascilin family with homology to FAS1.[4,5] It was originally characterized as a bone development protein,[6] a function reflected in the name periostin,[6] as well as its original name, osteoblast specific factor 2.[4] Periostin is expressed in multiple organs during normal development, tissue remodeling, wound healing, and response to injury (reviewed by Conway and colleagues[7] and Norris and colleagues[8]). It can be induced by several profibrotic stimuli[9] and has been demonstrated to regulate extracellular matrix (ECM) structure and organization through its ability to bind ECM (reviewed by Kii and Ito[10]) and promote collagen fibrillogenesis and cross-linking.[11] As a matricellular signaling protein, periostin can initiate fibrotic and nonfibrotic pathways in a cell-specific and tissue-specific manner.[9]

Periostin expression in normal and diseased tissue

Aside from its expression in bone and during development, periostin has been observed at sites of injury and regions of epithelial inflammation. In lung, the thickened subepithelial basement membrane of human bronchial asthma samples stained high for periostin[12,13] and subepithelial periostin levels at baseline in asthmatics negatively correlated with subsequent decline of lung function over 20 years.[14] Periostin expression has been observed in other Type 2 helper T-cells or type 2 (T2) immune diseases, including chronic rhinosinusitis with nasal polyps[15,16] and eosinophilic esophagitis.[17] In eosinophilic esophagitis, periostin diminished eosinophil chemotaxis and increased eosinophil adhesion to fibronectin, demonstrating a role for periostin in directly regulating eosinophil accumulation in T2 mucosal tissues.[17] Periostin expression in skin allergic disorders has been examined. Periostin is localized to the papillary dermis in normal and psoriatic skin but is expressed throughout the dermis of lesional skin in atopic dermatitis (AD),[18,19] implying increased IL-13 pathway activation in AD.

The dual function of periostin as an inflammatory and fibrotic pathway protein is reflected in the expression of periostin in areas of active lung fibrosis in idiopathic pulmonary fibrosis (IPF)[20] as well as in the lesional dermis of Systemic Sclerosis subjects, where it correlated with clinical disease activity.[21] In these diseases, fibrosis may be less IL-13 dependent, which may explain the lack of efficacy of anti–IL-13–directed therapy in IPF.[22,23]

Interleukin 4/interleukin 13 pathway activation and periostin induction

Periostin is down-stream of IL-4 and IL-13 signaling.[24] IL-13–induced or IL-4–induced periostin gene and protein expression is independent of transforming growth factor β.[12] The first studies to demonstrate periostin as a potential biomarker of T2 allergic asthma were 2 publications from Woodruff and colleagues. In a genome-wide microarray on epithelial brushings from asthmatics, smokers, and healthy controls, Woodruff and colleagues[13] showed that CLCA1, POSTN, and SERPINB2 were the top genes to distinguish allergic airway disease tissue from healthy. They also confirmed that periostin was released from IL-13–stimulated primary human airway epithelial cells grown in air-liquid interface (ALI). The investigators went on to show that these 3 genes could be used to subset asthmatics into T2 high or T2 low and that T2-high subjects had increased disease severity in terms of elevated airway hyper-responsiveness, IgE, mucus and eosinophils levels, and thickened basement membranes.[25] Silkoff and colleagues[26] examined gene induction from IL-13–treated human airway mucosal cells and identified CCL26 and POSTN as the top differentially expressed genes, although in this study *CCL26* was superior at segregating T2 asthmatics from non-T2 asthmatics. That periostin was the only gene common to these studies for identifying T2 asthmatics implies its high potential as an IL-13 pathway biomarker.

Circulating periostin levels

Because airway epithelial cells secrete periostin in a basal direction,[27] it is detectable in the blood, making it a potential biomarker candidate. The development of sensitive ELISAs measuring all splice forms of serum periostin (s-periostin) has allowed circulating levels to be quantified.[28,29] The performance of different periostin assays has been reviewed previously.[30] In serum, periostin is minimally elevated above levels in healthy subjects in general asthmatic populations.[28,31–34] Within T2-high asthma subjects (eg, by high fractional exhaled nitric oxide [FeNO], blood eosinophils, sputum eosinophils, tissue eosinophils, and IgE), however, the results are mixed. Jia and colleagues[29] found s-periostin level was the most sensitive marker to distinguish asthmatic subjects with a high lung eosinophil score from those with a low lung eosinophil score. Conversely, Wagener and colleagues[35] found no correlation between s-periostin and sputum eosinophilia, and s-periostin was not able to distinguish asthma subjects with eosinophilic inflammation from those with noneosinophilic inflammation. These differences may be due to the different assays used or the populations studied because Jia and colleagues used a more severe uncontrolled asthma cohort than Wagener and colleagues.

Elevated s-periostin levels are also associated with other allergic diseases. For example, s-periostin levels were elevated in chronic rhinosinusitis with nasal polyps subjects and could be used to distinguish subjects with and without polyps.[16,36,37] In AD, s-periostin levels correlated with disease severity and decreased after treatment.[18] Psoriatic subjects had lower levels of s-periostin than AD subjects but levels were higher than those in healthy controls.[18,38] In fibrotic indications, similar to what was seen with tissue expression, circulating periostin levels were elevated and s-periostin was predictive of clinical progression in IPF[20] and disease activity in systemic sclerosis,[21] indicating that s-periostin may be a prognostic biomarker for these diseases.

Dipeptidyl Peptidase-4

Background

DPP-4 is located on chromosome 2 and encoded by the *DPP4* gene. A 110-kDa glycoprotein, it is a serine protease in the S9 family of enzymes with the capability of cleaving amino-terminal dipeptides that have either L-alanine or L-proline at the penultimate position.[39,40] Alternative names for DPP-4 include DPP-IV, CD26, ADABP, ADCP2, and TP103.[41] DPP-4 can exist as membrane-bound and soluble protein. The soluble form is believed to originate from shedding of the membrane form into plasma.[39]

DPP-4 is more commonly recognized for its enzymatic activity, exemplified by its role in glucose metabolism for inactivating incretins, gastric inhibitory protein (GIP), and glucagon-like peptide-1 (GLP-1).[42] Another important enzymatic function of DPP-4 is in the metabolism of cytokines and chemokines (reviewed by Mortier and colleagues[43]). For example, with regard to asthma and allergy, CCL-11 (eotaxin) is a substrate for DPP-4.[39] This review focuses, however, on the gene and protein expression of DPP-4.

Dipeptidyl peptidase-4 expression in normal and diseased tissue

DPP-4 was shown to be ubiquitously expressed in kidney, liver, lung, and intestine, at endothelial and epithelial sites. It has also been shown to be expressed on immune cells including T cells, activated T cells, B cells, natural killer cells, and myeloid cells[39,44] and up-regulated on asthmatic CD4[+] T cells and invariant natural killer T cells.[44] As such, DPP-4 has been described as a surface antigen in T-cell activation and regulation, with potential involvement in various immune and neuroendocrine functions.[39,45]

In airway studies, the *DPP-4* gene was differentially expressed in nasal and bronchial transcriptomes from atopic asthmatics relative to nonatopic controls.[46] Immunostaining for DPP-4 protein was enhanced in airway bronchial epithelial cells (BECs) from steroid naïve relative to steroid-treated asthmatics.[47] These data are compatible with the observed effect of corticosteroids on serum DPP-4 (discussed later).

DPP-4 staining was increased in inflamed skin lesions from AD subjects compared with healthy nonatopic controls.[48] Moderate DPP-4 staining was seen in normal skin and localized to the dermis compared with AD skin, where both the dermis and epidermis were DPP-4 positive with particularly strong staining in the epidermis. The dermal DPP-4 staining in the AD skin, although lower than in the epidermis, was still elevated above the levels seen in healthy dermis. In contact dermatitis skin, DPP-4 staining was observed in the epidermis in a similar pattern to that observed in AD.[48]

Interleukin 4/interleukin 13 pathway activation and dipeptidyl peptidase-4 induction

DPP-4 has been shown to be induced by IL-13 in multiple models of asthma and allergy.[47,49–52] Similar to periostin, profibrotic molecules can also induce DPP-4 expression.[53] Furthermore, IL-13 gene expression positively correlated with *DPP4* mRNA expression in asthma patients on ICS and oral corticosteroids (OCS).[49,50] *DPP4* was also shown to be in the top 12 genes that positively correlated with *IL13* mRNA expression in transcriptomic studies of nasal epithelial cells and BECs from children with asthma.[46]

Circulating dipeptidyl peptidase-4 levels

Although early studies reported elevated serum DPP-4 levels in asthmatics relative to healthy subjects and no effect of ICS treatment,[44] more recent studies, with larger subject numbers, have contradicted both these observations. Serum DPP-4 protein concentrations were increased in patients with allergic asthma compared with healthy age-matched controls.[39] Furthermore, another study reported that healthy individuals had higher serum DPP-4 levels than severe asthmatics on ICS therapy.[54] Moreover, serum DPP-4 protein levels were lower in corticosteroid treated compared with corticosteroid-naïve patients with asthma.[47] Similarly, early correlations between serum DPP-4 levels and blood eosinophils have not reproduced in larger patient data sets, where no association of serum DPP-4 with IgE, forced expiratory volume in the first second of expiration (FEV$_1$), FeNO, and blood or sputum eosinophils was found.[55] Serum DPP-4 levels were inversely correlated with blood neutrophils in patients with severe airway disease.[55]

Summary

Periostin and DPP-4 show similarities in that they can both be induced by IL-13 and IL-4[24] and by other profibrotic stimuli.[9,53] This, however, may reduce their specificity as biomarkers of IL-13 pathway activity, which needs to be considered when using them for guiding treatment with anti–IL-13–directed therapies (because they may be elevated in patients with evidence of other concomitant fibrotic disease). Both periostin and DPP-4 gene and protein expression, however, are increased in patients with T2-associated diseases, including allergic asthma and AD, and both markers decrease with corticosteroid therapy. These data also imply that they are downstream of IL-13 pathway signaling in T2-associated diseases and can be markers of T2 disease and may, therefore, be candidate biomarkers of anti–IL-13–directed therapy.

DEMOGRAPHY/DISEASE

The ideal biomarker, as well as a measurable molecule that relates to disease status, should also be unaffected by other biological variables that could be present in the target patient population. Demographics, such as age and gender, or disease comorbidities may affect a biomarker and as such it is important to understand these relationships before a biomarker is used in the clinic.

Effects of Age and Gender on Periostin

Given its connection to bone metabolism, multiple studies have looked for gender or age differences in s-periostin levels. Overall, s-periostin was not different between men and women,[16,28,31,33,56] except in postmenopausal women with additional osteoporosis risk factors.[57] It has also been reported that s-periostin levels are equivalent in adult subjects across a range of ages[28,33,56,58] although 1 group reported higher s-periostin in subjects aged over 60, a presumed feedback loop in response to age-related bone catabolism.[31] Notably, s-periostin is elevated in teenage subjects relative to adults.[28,58] Furthermore, elevated levels of s-periostin in children ages 6 years to 11 years masked any increase due to allergic disease status.[58] Although unproved, the hypothesis is that active bone growth is the source of the raised s-periostin concentration in children and adolescents.[21,33] This may complicate the general use of periostin as a predictive biomarker for anti–IL-13–directed therapy, requiring different thresholds for defining s-periostin–high patients for therapy in adolescents compared with s-periostin–high patients for therapy in adults.

Effects of Body Mass Index Status on Periostin

Further potential confounders for use in predicting response to IL-13 pathway–directed therapy include BMI,[31,34] which was found to be inversely correlated with s-periostin levels independently of asthma status. Obesity is associated with cardiovascular and metabolic disease. Despite periostin's involvement in cardiac development, however, the association with cardiac complications has not been fully explored; a small study found no association with hypertension or heart disease.[33] Therefore, s-periostin may not have the equivalent strong association with metabolic disease and obesity that DPP-4 has (discussed later).

Effects of Cancer on Periostin

Both periostin and DPP-4 have been linked to cancer malignancies. Because both are pleiotropic proteins, this relationship could be the result of multiple mechanisms; epithelial mesenchymal transition, angiogenesis, and integrin activation in the case of periostin[59,60] or cell proliferation, migration, and adhesion for DPP-4.[61,62] The shared capacity to bind and organize ECM would also provide a direct effect, whereby these proteins may modify the tumor microenvironment and control metastasis. Despite this potential, these proteins may still have utility as biomarkers of IL-13 biology in T2 diseases. The prevalence of cancer is expected to be low in this population,[63,64] and, because cancer is usually an exclusion criterion in controlled clinical trials, this concern should not confound the interpretation of studies using periostin or DPP-4 as biomarkers to predict response.

Periostin Associations with Other Type 2 Biomarkers

A complete understanding of how a biomarker relates to other disease metrics is also important. In terms of a direct measure of airway inflammation, FeNO is an alternative noninvasive biomarker of T2 airway inflammation. FeNO is also downstream of IL-13 activation (reviewed by Ricciardolo and Silkoff[65]). Because both FeNO and periostin should reflect IL-13 pathway activity, they would be expected to correlate. Silkhoff and colleagues[26] showed that 80% of their periostin–high asthma subjects were also FeNO high. The lack of complete correlation likely reflects the incomplete selectivity of periostin (and FeNO for that matter) for IL-13. Other surrogate markers have been used to monitor T2 inflammation, including sputum or blood eosinophils. Weak, but significant, positive associations have been observed between serum and peripheral blood eosinophils.[29,31,33,66] This may be due, however, to the requirement for further segmentation of asthma patients with eosinophilic inflammation.[29,35] For example, although IL-13 can induce eosinophilic inflammation, there is a subpopulation of severe asthmatic patients with late-onset disease where IL-5 is the dominant cytokine for their eosinophilia[67] and these patients have low atopy. IgE, but not atopy, correlated with s-periostin levels.[31,33] Higher s-periostin concentrations were associated with elevated asthma exacerbation rate, but there have been mixed associations for s-periostin with changes in lung function (FEV_1 and forced vital capacity).[29,31,33,68]

Although the correlations are not perfect, these observations indicate the use of s-periostin as an alternative to FeNO, high IgE, and high blood eosinophils as a potential biomarker of T2 disease.

Effects of Corticosteroids on Periostin

Because many severe asthma subjects are on corticosteroids, the effect of this treatment on a biomarker must be assessed. Periostin gene expression was examined in airway epithelial cells from asthmatics prior to or after treatment with inhaled fluticasone.[13] Periostin gene expression was elevated in asthmatics (relative to healthy controls) and after fluticasone treatment *POSTN* expression was down-regulated relative to asthmatic subjects on placebo.[13] This finding was confirmed in vitro, where IL-13 stimulated *POSTN* expression in primary human airway epithelial cells cultured in ALI was inhibited by addition of dexamethasone or budesonide. Furthermore, high baseline expression of *POSTN* in airway epithelial brushings predicted improvements in FEV_1 at 4 weeks in the asthmatic subjects randomized to inhaled fluticasone.[13] When these data were reanalyzed using a 3-gene signature (*POSTN*, *CLCA1*, and *SERPINB2*) to define T2-high versus T2-low subjects, the T2-high cohorts showed significant improvement in FEV_1 at 4 weeks and 8 weeks of fluticasone treatment compared with T2-low subjects on fluticasone or placebo-treated asthmatics.[25] These findings demonstrate the sensitivity of periostin to corticosteroids but also its potential for guiding treatment of T2-high patients.

Effects of Age and Gender on Dipeptidyl Peptidase-4

There were 2 healthy population studies that reported that serum DPP-4 protein concentrations were higher in adolescents compared with adults.[54,69] Individuals ages 16 years to 21 years had the highest circulating DPP-4 levels, which subsequently decreased with advancing age.[54] With regard to differences in circulating DPP-4 protein among genders in the healthy population, 1 investigation reported that serum DPP-4 levels were higher in men compared with women.[54] In another study plasma and serum DPP-4 levels in healthy men trended slightly higher than healthy women but were not statistically different between genders in another study.[69] When matched for BMI status, male and female plasma DPP-4 levels were equivalent.[70]

Effects of Body Mass Index Status on Dipeptidyl Peptidase-4

There are conflicting data on the relationship of DPP-4 with BMI status. One study reported that serum DPP-4 levels did not change with BMI status,[54] whereas a second study showed plasma DPP-4 protein levels correlated with BMI higher in obese patients than normal weight individuals.[70]

Dipeptidyl Peptidase-4 Associations with Other Type 2 Biomarkers

There are few data available evaluating the relationship of serum DPP-4 with other T2 biomarkers. In 1 study, serum DPP-4 levels in asthmatics correlated with blood eosinophils[44] whereas in a more recent, larger study serum DPP-4 protein concentrations in asthma did not correlate with blood eosinophils or s-periostin.[50] *DPP4* mRNA expression from BECs and bronchial brushings from asthma patients on ICS and OCS, however, correlated positively with FeNO.[47,49,50] Because DPP-4 did not correlate with s-periostin, this suggests that DPP-4 may inform on different aspects of IL-13 pathway activation and, therefore, may provide an alternative biomarker for identifying patients to direct anti–IL-13 therapy.

Effects of Corticosteroids on Dipeptidyl Peptidase-4

In experimental studies, mometasone was shown to suppress IL-13 induced DPP-4 expression in BECs cultured in ALI.[51] In another study, DPP-4 protein was shown to be reduced in serum and BECs, along with mRNA expression in bronchial epithelium, from patients with asthma on ICS compared with steroid-naïve asthmatics.[47] Other studies have also demonstrated that serum DPP-4 protein levels were reduced in asthma patients with severe disease who were on corticosteroid regimens compared with healthy controls.[54]

These observations indicate that DPP-4, like IL-13, can be modulated by corticosteroid treatment. It is unknown, however, whether this is a direct effect of corticosteroids on DPP-4 expression or a downstream effect due to reduction in IL-13 expression. Although it has been shown that both periostin and DPP-4 can be modulated by corticosteroids, the use of biologic anti–IL-13–directed therapies would be used in severe uncontrolled asthma patients who demonstrate evidence of raised serum concentrations of these molecules despite receiving high-dosage corticosteroid therapy.

Other Drugs That May Have an Impact on Circulating Dipeptidyl Peptidase-4 Concentrations

As discussed previously, DPP-4 is involved in glucose metabolism by inactivating incretins, GIP and GLP-1, and is a target for treatment of patients with T2 diabetes by inhibiting its enzymatic activity.[42] The impact of DPP-4 inhibitors has been studied for effects on DPP-4 protein levels in serum. One study showed that there was an increase in plasma DPP-4 levels in diabetic patients treated with sitagliptin compared with predose levels.[71] Hence, the use of DPP-4 inhibitors may also confound the potential to determine protein DPP-4 concentrations for anti–IL-13–directed therapy.

Summary

When comparing these biomarkers by demographic characteristics and other T2 markers, differences begin to be seen between them. Both markers show similarities in relationship of serum levels with age, higher in adolescents than adults. This is where the similarities, however, seem to end. Periostin was shown to inversely correlate with BMI, whereas DPP-4 demonstrated either no association or a positive correlation with BMI. This may be due to DPP-4 also being a marker of metabolic disease, therefore reflecting glucose metabolism activity.

Of particular interest is the difference in the relationship of these biomarkers with other T2 biomarkers. Serum levels of periostin have shown positive relationships with FeNO, blood eosinophils, and serum IgE. Serum levels of DPP-4 have shown no correlation with blood eosinophils or s-periostin. Local expression of DPP-4 in the airway, however, did show a relationship with FeNO in asthmatics. It is possible that serum DPP-4 may represent other components of IL-13 biology or that serum levels of DPP-4 are indicative of both T2 disease activity and glucose metabolism activity, whereas local airway expression may be more reflective of local T2 pathway activation. These differences may have an impact on periostin's and DPP-4's capacity to predict response to anti–IL-13–directed therapy.

SERUM PERIOSTIN AND DIPEPTIDYL PEPTIDASE-4 TO DIRECT TREATMENT IN ASTHMA AND ALLERGIC DISEASE
Studies with Serum Periostin

Because asthma is a heterogeneous disease, a biomarker may be required to identify those patients with evidence of IL-13 pathway activation to direct anti–IL-13–therapy. Lebrikizumab, tralokinumab, and dupilumab are 3 monoclonal antibodies that can inhibit the IL-13 pathway in asthma and allergic disease.

Lebrikizumab is a humanized IgG_4 monoclonal antibody that specifically binds to IL-13 and inhibits its function.[72] In an initial phase 2 randomized, placebo-controlled, clinical study conducted in moderate to severe uncontrolled asthmatic patients taking inhaled corticosteroids, lebrikizumab was dosed monthly for 6 months. In this study, the primary endpoint was change in prebronchodilator FEV_1 from baseline to week 12. In the total study population, treatment with lebrikizumab demonstrated a statistically significant improvement in FEV_1 compared with placebo at week 12. When patients were subdivided into those with high or low s-periostin at baseline (the cutoff value was the study population median concentration of periostin), however, there was a greater effect on improvement in FEV_1 at week 12 compared with placebo in those with high compared with those with low s-periostin levels.[73] This initial clinical study confirmed the hypothesis that patients with evidence of IL-13 pathway activation would have greater benefit from anti–IL-13 therapy and further that s-periostin might be useful as a biomarker to identify such patients. Two further dose-ranging studies in patients with uncontrolled asthma despite using medium-dose to high-dose ICS plus a second controller medication demonstrated greater efficacy in s-periostin–high compared with s-periostin–low patients, this time on a primary endpoint of rate of asthma exacerbations during a median treatment duration of 24 weeks. This was a striking difference of a 60% reduction in s-periostin–high patients compared with a 5% reduction in s-periostin–low patients.[68] In a dose-ranging study in mild asthmatics not taking inhaled corticosteroids, where the primary endpoint was change from baseline in FEV_1, there was a numerically greater but clinically and statistically insignificant change in FEV_1 compared with placebo and there was no difference when subgrouping patients by baseline s-periostin levels.[22] This outcome may be because the patient population in this study was too mild to detect changes in lung function.

The lebrikizumab asthma program culminated in 2 phase 3 studies conducted in adult, uncontrolled severe asthmatics on high-dosage ICS plus at least 1 additional controller medication, LAVOLTA I and LAVOLTA II. These studies consisted of a 52-week treatment period with 2 dose regimens of lebrikizumab compared with placebo and with patients stratified to treatment based on baseline s-periostin concentration. The primary endpoint was rate of exacerbations; however, the primary population for analysis was biomarker-high patients, defined as periostin greater than or equal to 50 ng/mL or blood eosinophils greater than or equal to 300 cells/μL. Although LAVOLTA I demonstrated a statistically and clinically meaningful improvement on annual asthma exacerbation rate (AAER) compared with placebo with both lebrikizumab doses, LAVOLTA II missed statistical significance. In the secondary analyses, both studies demonstrated statistically and clinically significant improvements in asthma exacerbation rate compared with placebo in patients who were s-periostin high but inconsistent efficacy in patients who were s-periostin low.[74] Extending the primary analysis population to include patients with high blood eosinophil or high s-periostin may have included a more heterogenous group of patients, because although IL-13 can induce eosinophilia, there are patients with high blood eosinophils with late-onset disease who are more dependent on IL-5 and less atopic.[67] The utility of s-periostin to predict efficacy with anti–IL-13 therapy was confirmed in these trials.

Tralokinumab is a human IgG_4 monoclonal antibody that neutralizes IL-13.[75] In an initial phase 2a study in patients with moderate to severe asthma and a primary endpoint of change from baseline in mean Asthma Control Questionnaire (ACQ)-6 score, a 12-week treatment period with tralokinumab showed no statistically significant difference compared with placebo. In a subgroup of patients, however, where sputum IL-13 levels were measured, patients with high sputum IL-13 showed greater changes in ACQ-6 and FEV_1 compared with those with low sputum IL-13. A later phase 2b, randomized, placebo-controlled study investigating 2 dosing regimens of tralokinumab in adult patients with severe uncontrolled asthma with treatment for 1 year and a primary endpoint of AAER evaluated the concept of s-periostin to identify patients who would gain benefit from treatment with tralokinumab.[76] There was no difference between tralokinumab treatment and placebo on exacerbation rate reduction or secondary endpoints of change in ACQ-6 or Asthma Quality of Life Questionnaire (AQLQ) in the intention-to-treat (ITT) population.[76] At week 52, however, there was a significant increase in FEV_1 compared with placebo in patients receiving tralokinumab every 2 weeks.

Subgrouping patients by s-periostin high and s-periostin low (using study population median concentration as a cutpoint), showed a numerically greater but statistically nonsignificant reduction in exacerbation rate in patients treated with tralokinumab compared with the effect in the ITT study population in patients with high s-periostin at baseline but not in patients with low s-periostin. Increases in FEV_1 at week 52 were similar between patients in the high-periostin and low-periostin subgroups receiving tralokinumab versus placebo. Improvement in ACQ-6 was greater in s-periostin–high patients compared with s-periostin–low patients but not statistically significant, and there was no difference in AQLQ improvement.

In a post hoc analysis with further subsetting, it was shown in a subgroup of patients not receiving chronic OCS therapy and with airway reversibility at baseline that there were further numerical and statistically significant improvements in exacerbation rate, FEV_1, and ACQ-6 but not AQLQ in patients with high s-periostin but not low s-periostin. These studies with tralokinumab again highlighted the need for directed therapy for asthma patients based on a biomarker to identify those patients with evidence of IL-13 pathway activation.

The phase 3 program with tralokinumab included 2 pivotal studies in patients with severe uncontrolled asthma, despite treatment with ICS plus long-acting β_2-agonists, with demonstrated postbronchodilator reversibility to short-acting β_2-agonists and not on chronic OCS therapy. STRATOS 1 (NCT02161757) and STRATOS 2 (NCT02194699) were both designed with the primary outcome of annual AAER.[77] Patients were stratified at randomization in both studies by baseline s-periostin levels (<16.44 ng/mL or greater than or equal to 16.44 ng/mL; corresponding to the median value observed in previous studies). The studies were run concurrently but analyzed sequentially. The aim was to use the results from STRATOS 1 to identify a target population with enhanced response to treatment with tralokinumab based on baseline levels of biomarkers associated with IL-13 pathway activation, including s-periostin, DPP-4, FeNO, and total serum IgE. The results from STRATOS 1 determined the biomarker-positive population to be assessed in STRATOS 2.[77] AstraZeneca (Cambridge, U.K.) has announced that STRATOS 1 and STRATOS 2 both failed to achieve their respective primary endpoints.[78,79] In STRATOS 1, the primary endpoint of a significant reduction in AAER in the overall study population was not met, but it was reported that a clinically relevant reduction in AAER was observed in a subpopulation of patients with an elevated biomarker associated with increased IL-13 activity, which would be the focus for the analysis of STRATOS 2.[78] The later announcement of STRATOS 2 reported that the biomarker selected for the subpopulation analysis was patients with elevated FeNO, but that the primary endpoint was not met.[79] At the time of writing this review, no data have been reported on the performance of s-periostin and serum DPP-4 in these studies.

Dupilumab is a fully human monoclonal antibody directed against the IL-4 receptor alpha subunit and inhibits both IL-4 and IL-13 signaling.[80] In a phase 2b study in uncontrolled, moderate to severe asthmatics, where the primary analysis population was patients with blood eosinophils greater than or equal to 300 cells/µL, dupilumab showed statistically significant improvements in lung function, exacerbation rate, ACQ-5, and AQLQ. Similar changes were also observed, however, in the total study population and patients with blood eosinophils less than 300 cells/µL, suggesting efficacy in a wide range of patients. A post hoc analysis also showed that there was efficacy in patients who were s-periostin high and s-periostin low, although efficacy was numerically greater in those patients who were s-periostin high.[81] These findings were in contrast to the data with the monoclonal antibodies that target IL-13, suggesting that combined targeting of IL-4 and IL-13 may have a broader therapeutic role in severe asthma.

Dupilumab has also demonstrated efficacy in AD and nasal polyposis, but there has been no evaluation of efficacy by biomarkers in these diseases.[82,83]

Finally, the effect of s-periostin to predict efficacy in treating patients with omalizumab has also been evaluated. Omalizumab is a humanized IgG1κ monoclonal antibody that specifically binds to free human IgE.[84] In patients with uncontrolled severe persistent allergic asthma, analyses were performed evaluating treatment effects to T2 biomarkers that included baseline s-periostin. After 48 weeks of omalizumab, reductions in protocol-defined exacerbations were greater in high s-periostin versus low s-periostin.[85] Therefore, periostin may also be a biomarker for other T2-directed therapies. This is perhaps not surprising, because IL-13 can direct class switching of immunoglobulin production to IgE from B cells.[1]

Studies with Serum Dipeptidyl Peptidase-4

Asthma

Currently, available data on the potential utility of DPP-4 as a predictive biomarker for anti–IL-13 treatment in asthma is limited to the same phase 2b study with tralokinumab that also investigated the utility of s-periostin (described previously[76]). As discussed previously, although serum DPP-4 concentrations were lower in patients with asthma than healthy volunteers, some patients had high concentrations despite corticosteroid therapy. Therefore, a post hoc analysis was conducted that hypothesized elevated serum DPP-4, despite high corticosteroid dosages, may identify patients who benefit from tralokinumab.

Similar to results observed subsetting by s-periostin levels, there were greater reductions in annual exacerbation rate in DPP-4 high than DPP-4 low; however, these reductions were not significant compared with placebo. Unlike that observed by s-periostin subgrouping, numerically greater and significant improvements in prebronchodilator FEV_1 were seen in the DPP-4–high subset but not in DPP-4–low subset. Furthermore, in contrast to the high s-periostin group, numerically greater and statistically significant improvements in ACQ-6 and AQLQ compared with placebo at week 52 were seen in patients receiving tralokinumab in the DPP-4–high subgroup. In the DPP-4–low subset, all changes were of a lower magnitude than the DPP-4–high subgroup and none was statistically significant.

Further subsetting of patients investigated serum DPP-4–high and DPP-4–low patients receiving tralokinumab with airway reversibility at baseline but not receiving long-term OCS. This post hoc analysis revealed further improvements in the magnitude of reduction of AAER rate versus placebo, but again these did not achieve statistical significance, probably due to the low subject number.

Within this subset there were also further improvements in FEV_1, ACQ-6, and AQLQ in those who were DPP-4 high, which achieved statistical significance. In the DPP-4–low group, again changes were small and no outcomes achieved statistical significance. The data in those who were DPP-4 high are again in contrast to those who were s-periostin high, which showed no significant improvement in AQLQ.

Atopic dermatitis

Currently, available data on the potential utility of DPP-4 as a predictive biomarker for anti–IL-13 treatment in adults with moderate to severe AD is limited to a single phase 2b study with tralokinumab.[86] The coprimary endpoints were change from baseline in total Eczema Area and Severity Index (EASI) and percentage of Investigator's Global Assessment (IGA) responders (patients achieving an IGA of 0 or 1 and at least a 2-grade reduction from baseline) at week 12. Tralokinumab at 150 mg and 300 mg in the ITT population significantly reduced total EASI from baseline and a greater number of patients had an IGA response of 0 or 1 compared with placebo.

In an exploratory analysis, patients were subgrouped by median baseline serum DPP-4 to DPP-4 high and DPP-4 low. In summary, DPP-4–high moderate to severe AD patients demonstrated significant efficacy in both primary endpoints compared with placebo with effect sizes greater than in the ITT population at week 12 after treatment with 300 mg tralokinumab. No significant differences in either primary endpoint was observed for the DPP-4–low subgroup. These data suggest serum DPP-4 may also serve as a predictive biomarker for AD patients who may benefit from tralokinumab treatment.

Summary

Subgrouping severe asthma patients by baseline levels of s-periostin or serum DPP-4 into biomarker high and low subpopulations demonstrated greater efficacy on clinical efficacy endpoints in the biomarker high subgroup compared with biomarker low for treatment with anti–IL-13 monoclonal antibodies. For s-periostin, this was despite different assay formats that were used for trials with lebrikizumab[74] and tralokinumab.[76]

In the phase 2b clinical study with tralokinumab that explored the use of both s-periostin and serum DPP-4, there were differences in how each biomarker performed to predict efficacy response. In this study, s-periostin–high patients showed numerically greater magnitude of effect on exacerbation rate reduction but lower magnitudes of effect on improvements in FEV_1 and ACQ-6 and little to no effect on AQLQ compared with the efficacy responses in the subgroup of patients who were serum DPP-4 high. This may indicate that s-periostin and DPP-4 have different biology associated with IL-13 activation and therefore can inform on different efficacy endpoints. The results using s-periostin to predict efficacy with omalizumab (anti-IgE) therapy also indicate that s-periostin may be a biomarker for predicting response to other T2-directed therapies. Furthermore, the data with serum DPP-4 in AD also suggest these biomarkers may have utility in other T2 diseases as well as asthma.

OVERALL SUMMARY

Periostin and DPP-4 are both induced by the T2 cytokines IL-4 and IL-13 and have increased local expression in T2 disease tissue, including lung, nasal, and skin. Furthermore, they are measurable in serum, supporting their potential for practical application in the clinical setting. Both markers share similar factors that can potentially confound their specificity as markers of T2 inflammation with both induced by profibrotic factors and also being increased in the serum of adolescents compared with adults.

There are also striking differences between these 2 serum biomarkers, however, particularly with respect to their relationship with other T2 biomarkers. In general, periostin shows correlations with other T2 markers, unlike DPP-4 that shows no relationship. Furthermore, there is no correlation between s-periostin and serum DPP-4.

In clinical trials of severe, uncontrolled asthma, periostin has consistently demonstrated enhanced efficacy of anti–IL-13 therapy in patients with high serum levels. The available data with serum DPP-4 are more limited, restricted to 1 study with tralokinumab in asthma and 1 in AD. Patients with high DPP-4, however, also showed enhanced efficacy to treatment with tralokinumab in both asthma and AD.

High s-periostin levels also showed enhanced efficacy to treatment with omalizumab, indicating that periostin may also have application as a more general marker of T2 inflammatory disease.

The failure of lebrikizumab and tralokinumab to meet the primary endpoints in their respective phase 3 asthma programs may suggest there is little need for biomarkers for anti–IL-13–directed therapy in asthma, especially because dupilumab has shown efficacy in s-periostin–high and s-periostin–low subgroups. Despite this, they may still be of value in understanding the pathologic mechanisms of severe asthma.

REFERENCES

1. Hershey GK. IL-13 receptors and signaling pathways: an evolving web. J Allergy Clin Immunol 2003;111(4):677–90 [quiz: 691].
2. Saha SK, Berry MA, Parker D, et al. Increased sputum and bronchial biopsy IL-13 expression in severe asthma. J Allergy Clin Immunol 2008;121(3):685–91.
3. Cai F, Choy DF, Brumm J, et al. Serum IL-13 is a peripheral biomarker for type 2 asthma. Eur Respir J 2015.
4. Takeshita S, Kikuno R, Tezuka K, et al. Osteoblast-specific factor 2: cloning of a putative bone adhesion protein with homology with the insect protein fasciclin I. Biochem J 1993;294(Pt 1):271–8.
5. POSTN periostin [Homo sapiens (human)] - Gene - NCBI. 2018. Available at: https://www.ncbi.nlm.nih.gov/pubmed/.
6. Horiuchi K, Amizuka N, Takeshita S, et al. Identification and characterization of a novel protein, periostin, with restricted expression to periosteum and periodontal

ligament and increased expression by transforming growth factor beta. J Bone Miner Res 1999;14(7):1239–49.

7. Conway SJ, Izuhara K, Kudo Y, et al. The role of periostin in tissue remodeling across health and disease. Cell Mol Life Sci 2014;71(7):1279–88.

8. Norris RA, Moreno-Rodriguez R, Hoffman S, et al. The many facets of the matricelluar protein periostin during cardiac development, remodeling, and pathophysiology. J Cell Commun Signal 2009;3(3–4):275–86.

9. Rosselli-Murai LK, Almeida LO, Zagni C, et al. Periostin responds to mechanical stress and tension by activating the MTOR signaling pathway. PLoS One 2013; 8(12):e83580.

10. Kii I, Ito H. Periostin and its interacting proteins in the construction of extracellular architectures. Cell Mol Life Sci 2017;74(23):4269–77.

11. Maruhashi T, Kii I, Saito M, et al. Interaction between periostin and BMP-1 promotes proteolytic activation of lysyl oxidase. J Biol Chem 2010;285(17): 13294–303.

12. Takayama G, Arima K, Kanaji T, et al. Periostin: a novel component of subepithelial fibrosis of bronchial asthma downstream of IL-4 and IL-13 signals. J Allergy Clin Immunol 2006;118(1):98–104.

13. Woodruff PG, Boushey HA, Dolganov GM, et al. Genome-wide profiling identifies epithelial cell genes associated with asthma and with treatment response to corticosteroids. Proc Natl Acad Sci U S A 2007;104(40):15858–63.

14. Kanemitsu Y, Ito I, Niimi A, et al. Osteopontin and periostin are associated with a 20-year decline of pulmonary function in patients with asthma. Am J Respir Crit Care Med 2014;190(4):472–4.

15. Stankovic KM, Goldsztein H, Reh DD, et al. Gene expression profiling of nasal polyps associated with chronic sinusitis and aspirin-sensitive asthma. Laryngoscope 2008;118(5):881–9.

16. Maxfield AZ, Landegger LD, Brook CD, et al. Periostin as a biomarker for nasal polyps in chronic rhinosinusitis. Otolaryngol Head Neck Surg 2018;158(1):181–6.

17. Blanchard C, Mingler MK, McBride M, et al. Periostin facilitates eosinophil tissue infiltration in allergic lung and esophageal responses. Mucosal Immunol 2008; 1(4):289–96.

18. Kou K, Okawa T, Yamaguchi Y, et al. Periostin levels correlate with disease severity and chronicity in patients with atopic dermatitis. Br J Dermatol 2014; 171(2):283–91.

19. Zhou HM, Wang J, Elliott C, et al. Spatiotemporal expression of periostin during skin development and incisional wound healing: lessons for human fibrotic scar formation. J Cell Commun Signal 2010;4(2):99–107.

20. Naik PK, Bozyk PD, Bentley JK, et al. Periostin promotes fibrosis and predicts progression in patients with idiopathic pulmonary fibrosis. Am J Physiol Lung Cell Mol Physiol 2012;303(12):L1046–56.

21. Yamaguchi Y, Ono J, Masuoka M, et al. Serum periostin levels are correlated with progressive skin sclerosis in patients with systemic sclerosis. Br J Dermatol 2013; 168(4):717–25.

22. Noonan M, Korenblat P, Mosesova S, et al. Dose-ranging study of lebrikizumab in asthmatic patients not receiving inhaled steroids. J Allergy Clin Immunol 2013; 132(3):567–74.e12.

23. Parker JM, Glaspole IN, Lancaster LH, et al. A phase 2 randomized controlled study of tralokinumab in subjects with idiopathic pulmonary fibrosis. Am J Respir Crit Care Med 2018;197(1):94–103.

24. Yuyama N, Davies DE, Akaiwa M, et al. Analysis of novel disease-related genes in bronchial asthma. Cytokine 2002;19(6):287–96.

25. Woodruff PG, Modrek B, Choy DF, et al. T-helper type 2-driven inflammation defines major subphenotypes of asthma. Am J Respir Crit Care Med 2009;180(5): 388–95.

26. Silkoff PE, Laviolette M, Singh D, et al. Identification of airway mucosal type 2 inflammation by using clinical biomarkers in asthmatic patients. J Allergy Clin Immunol 2017;140(3):710–9.

27. Sidhu SS, Yuan S, Innes AL, et al. Roles of epithelial cell-derived periostin in TGF-beta activation, collagen production, and collagen gel elasticity in asthma. Proc Natl Acad Sci U S A 2010;107(32):14170–5.

28. Jeanblanc NM, Hemken PM, Datwyler MJ, et al. Development of a new ARCHITECT automated periostin immunoassay. Clin Chim Acta 2017;464:228–35.

29. Jia G, Erickson RW, Choy DF, et al. Periostin is a systemic biomarker of eosinophilic airway inflammation in asthmatic patients. J Allergy Clin Immunol 2012; 130(3):647–54.e10.

30. Arron JR, Izuhara K. Asthma biomarkers: what constitutes a 'gold standard'? Thorax 2015;70(2):105–7.

31. James A, Janson C, Malinovschi A, et al. Serum periostin relates to type-2 inflammation and lung function in asthma: data from the large population-based cohort Swedish GA(2)LEN. Allergy 2017;72(11):1753–60.

32. Fingleton J, Braithwaite I, Travers J, et al. Serum periostin in obstructive airways disease. Eur Respir J 2016;47(5):1383–91.

33. Caswell-Smith R, Hosking A, Cripps T, et al. Reference ranges for serum periostin in a population without asthma or chronic obstructive pulmonary disease. Clin Exp Allergy 2016;46(10):1303–14.

34. Caswell-Smith R, Cripps T, Charles T, et al. Day-time variation of serum periostin in asthmatic adults treated with ICS/LABA and adults without asthma. Allergy Asthma Clin Immunol 2017;13:8.

35. Wagener AH, de Nijs SB, Lutter R, et al. External validation of blood eosinophils, FE(NO) and serum periostin as surrogates for sputum eosinophils in asthma. Thorax 2015;70(2):115–20.

36. Jonstam K, Westman M, Holtappels G, et al. Serum periostin, IgE, and SE-IgE can be used as biomarkers to identify moderate to severe chronic rhinosinusitis with nasal polyps. J Allergy Clin Immunol 2017;140(6):1705–8.e3.

37. Asano T, Kanemitsu Y, Takemura M, et al. Serum periostin as a biomarker for comorbid chronic rhinosinusitis in patients with asthma. Ann Am Thorac Soc 2017; 14(5):667–75.

38. Arima K, Ohta S, Takagi A, et al. Periostin contributes to epidermal hyperplasia in psoriasis common to atopic dermatitis. Allergol Int 2015;64(1):41–8.

39. Klemann C, Wagner L, Stephan M, et al. Cut to the chase: a review of CD26/dipeptidyl peptidase-4's (DPP4) entanglement in the immune system. Clin Exp Immunol 2016;185(1):1–21.

40. Nieto-Fontarigo JJ, Gonzalez-Barcala FJ, San Jose E, et al. CD26 and asthma: a comprehensive review. Clin Rev Allergy Immunol 2016. [Epub ahead of print].

41. DPP4 dipeptidyl peptidase 4 [Homo sapiens (human)] - Gene - NCBI. 2018. Available at: https://www.ncbi.nlm.nih.gov/pubmed/.

42. Lambeir AM, Durinx C, Scharpe S, et al. Dipeptidyl-peptidase IV from bench to bedside: an update on structural properties, functions, and clinical aspects of the enzyme DPP IV. Crit Rev Clin Lab Sci 2003;40(3):209–94.

43. Mortier A, Gouwy M, Van Damme J, et al. CD26/dipeptidylpeptidase IV-chemokine interactions: double-edged regulation of inflammation and tumor biology. J Leukoc Biol 2016;99(6):955–69.
44. Lun SW, Wong CK, Ko FW, et al. Increased expression of plasma and CD4+ T lymphocyte costimulatory molecule CD26 in adult patients with allergic asthma. J Clin Immunol 2007;27(4):430–7.
45. Frerker N, Raber K, Bode F, et al. Phenotyping of congenic dipeptidyl peptidase 4 (DP4) deficient Dark Agouti (DA) rats suggests involvement of DP4 in neuro-, endocrine, and immune functions. Clin Chem Lab Med 2009;47(3):275–87.
46. Poole A, Urbanek C, Eng C, et al. Dissecting childhood asthma with nasal transcriptomics distinguishes subphenotypes of disease. J Allergy Clin Immunol 2014;133(3):670–8.e12.
47. Shiobara T, Chibana K, Watanabe T, et al. Dipeptidyl peptidase-4 is highly expressed in bronchial epithelial cells of untreated asthma and it increases cell proliferation along with fibronectin production in airway constitutive cells. Respir Res 2016;17:28.
48. Tasic T, Baumer W, Schmiedl A, et al. Dipeptidyl peptidase IV (DPP4) deficiency increases Th1-driven allergic contact dermatitis. Clin Exp Allergy 2011;41(8):1098–107.
49. Ranade K, Kuziora M, Pham T-H, et al. Dipeptidyl peptidase-4 (DPP-4) may predict response to tralokinumab in patients with asthma. Eur Respir J 2016;48(suppl 60).
50. Ranade K, Pham T-H, Damera G, et al. Dipeptidyl peptidase-4 (DPP-4) is a novel predictive biomarker for the investigational anti-IL-13 targeted therapy tralokinumab. Am J Respir Crit Care Med 2016;193:A4332.
51. Chibana K, Shiobara T, Watanabe T, et al. Regulation of dipeptydyl peptidase-4 (DPP4) expression in bronchial epithelial cells (BECs). Am J Respir Crit Care Med 2016;193:A1467.
52. Zhang Y, Urbanek C, Burchard EG, et al. The asthma biomarker dipeptidyl peptidase 4 (DPP4) is IL-13 inducible in airway epithelial cells and inhibits rhinovirus infection. Am J Respir Crit Care Med 2014;189:A4875.
53. Xin Y, Wang X, Zhu M, et al. Expansion of CD26 positive fibroblast population promotes keloid progression. Exp Cell Res 2017;356(1):104–13.
54. Hemken PM, Jeanblanc NM, Rae T, et al. Development and analytical performance of a new ARCHITECT automated dipeptidyl peptidase-4 immunoassay. Pract Lab Med 2017;9:58–68.
55. James A, Kolmert J, Knowles R, et al. Lack of association between circulating dipeptidyl peptidase-4 and type 2 biomarkers in asthma; data from U-BIOPRED and BIOAIR cohorts. Eur Respir J 2016;48(suppl 60).
56. Walsh JS, Gossiel F, Scott JR, et al. Effect of age and gender on serum periostin: relationship to cortical measures, bone turnover and hormones. Bone 2017;99:8–13.
57. Chapurlat RD, Confavreux CB. Novel biological markers of bone: from bone metabolism to bone physiology. Rheumatology (Oxford) 2016;55(10):1714–25.
58. Inoue Y, Izuhara K, Ohta S, et al. No increase in the serum periostin level is detected in elementary school-age children with allergic diseases. Allergol Int 2015;64(3):289–90.
59. Idolazzi L, Ridolo E, Fassio A, et al. Periostin: the bone and beyond. Eur J Intern Med 2017;38:12–6.
60. Morra L, Moch H. Periostin expression and epithelial-mesenchymal transition in cancer: a review and an update. Virchows Arch 2011;459(5):465–75.

61. Beckenkamp A, Davies S, Willig JB, et al. DPPIV/CD26: a tumor suppressor or a marker of malignancy? Tumour Biol 2016;37(6):7059–73.

62. Cordero OJ, Salgado FJ, Nogueira M. On the origin of serum CD26 and its altered concentration in cancer patients. Cancer Immunol Immunother 2009;58(11): 1723–47.

63. Gonzalez-Perez A, Fernandez-Vidaurre C, Rueda A, et al. Cancer incidence in a general population of asthma patients. Pharmacoepidemiol Drug Saf 2006;15(2): 131–8.

64. Rosenberger A, Bickeboller H, McCormack V, et al. Asthma and lung cancer risk: a systematic investigation by the International Lung Cancer Consortium. Carcinogenesis 2012;33(3):587–97.

65. Ricciardolo FLM, Silkoff PE. Perspectives on exhaled nitric oxide. J Breath Res 2017;11(4):047104.

66. Matsusaka M, Kabata H, Fukunaga K, et al. Phenotype of asthma related with high serum periostin levels. Allergol Int 2015;64(2):175–80.

67. de Groot JC, Ten Brinke A, Bel EH. Management of the patient with eosinophilic asthma: a new era begins. ERJ Open Res 2015;1(1) [pii:00024-2015].

68. Hanania NA, Noonan M, Corren J, et al. Lebrikizumab in moderate-to-severe asthma: pooled data from two randomised placebo-controlled studies. Thorax 2015;70(8):748–56.

69. Durinx C, Neels H, Van der Auwera JC, et al. Reference values for plasma dipeptidyl-peptidase IV activity and their association with other laboratory parameters. Clin Chem Lab Med 2001;39(2):155–9.

70. Stengel A, Goebel-Stengel M, Teuffel P, et al. Obese patients have higher circulating protein levels of dipeptidyl peptidase IV. Peptides 2014;61:75–82.

71. Makdissi A, Ghanim H, Vora M, et al. Sitagliptin exerts an antinflammatory action. J Clin Endocrinol Metab 2012;97(9):3333–41.

72. Ultsch M, Bevers J, Nakamura G, et al. Structural basis of signaling blockade by anti-IL-13 antibody Lebrikizumab. J Mol Biol 2013;425(8):1330–9.

73. Corren J, Lemanske RF, Hanania NA, et al. Lebrikizumab treatment in adults with asthma. N Engl J Med 2011;365(12):1088–98.

74. Hanania NA, Korenblat P, Chapman KR, et al. Efficacy and safety of lebrikizumab in patients with uncontrolled asthma (LAVOLTA I and LAVOLTA II): replicate, phase 3, randomised, double-blind, placebo-controlled trials. Lancet Respir Med 2016;4(10):781–96.

75. May RD, Monk PD, Cohen ES, et al. Preclinical development of CAT-354, an IL-13 neutralizing antibody, for the treatment of severe uncontrolled asthma. Br J Pharmacol 2012;166(1):177–93.

76. Brightling CE, Chanez P, Leigh R, et al. Efficacy and safety of tralokinumab in patients with severe uncontrolled asthma: a randomised, double-blind, placebo-controlled, phase 2b trial. Lancet Respir Med 2015;3(9):692–701.

77. Panettieri RA, Brightling C, Sjobring U, et al. STRATOS 1 and 2: considerations in clinical trial design for a fully human monoclonal antibody in severe asthma. Clin Investig (Lond) 2015;5(8):701–11.

78. AstraZeneca provides update on STRATOS 1 phase III trial of tralokinumab in severe, uncontrolled asthma. 2018. Available at: https://www.astrazeneca.com/media-centre/press-releases/2017/astrazeneca-provides-update-on-stratos-1-phase-iii-trial-of-tralokinumab-in-severe-uncontrolled-asthma-100517.html.

79. AstraZeneca provides update on tralokinumab phase III programme in severe, uncontrolled asthma. 2018. Available at: https://www.astrazeneca.com/media-

centre/press-releases/2017/astrazeneca-provides-update-on-tralokinumab-phase-iii-programme-in-severe-uncontrolled-asthma-01112017.html.

80. Wenzel S, Castro M, Corren J, et al. Dupilumab efficacy and safety in adults with uncontrolled persistent asthma despite use of medium-to-high-dose inhaled corticosteroids plus a long-acting beta2 agonist: a randomised double-blind placebo-controlled pivotal phase 2b dose-ranging trial. Lancet 2016;388(10039): 31–44.

81. Wenzel S, Swanson B, Teper A, et al. Dupilumab reduces severe exacerbations in periostin-high and periostin-low asthma patients. Paper presented at: European Respiratory Society. 2016.

82. Bachert C, Mannent L, Naclerio RM, et al. Effect of subcutaneous dupilumab on nasal polyp burden in patients with chronic sinusitis and nasal polyposis: a randomized clinical trial. JAMA 2016;315(5):469–79.

83. Simpson EL, Bieber T, Guttman-Yassky E, et al. Two phase 3 trials of dupilumab versus placebo in atopic dermatitis. N Engl J Med 2016;375(24):2335–48.

84. Presta LG, Lahr SJ, Shields RL, et al. Humanization of an antibody directed against IgE. J Immunol 1993;151(5):2623–32.

85. Hanania NA, Wenzel S, Rosen K, et al. Exploring the effects of omalizumab in allergic asthma: an analysis of biomarkers in the EXTRA study. Am J Respir Crit Care Med 2013;187(8):804–11.

86. Wollenberg AH, Howell MD, Guttman-Yassky E, et al. A phase 2b dose-ranging efficacy and safety study of tralokinumab in adult patients with moderate to severe atopic dermatitis (AD). J Am Acad Dermatol 2017;76(6):AB20.

The Role of Neutrophils in Asthma

Reynold A. Panettieri Jr, MD

KEYWORDS

- Steroid insensitivity • Irreversible airway obstruction • Severe asthma • Immunocyte
- Airway remodeling • Intrinsic asthma

KEY POINTS

- Although asthma defines a syndrome associated with airway inflammation, heterogeneity exists concerning the type of inflammation that modulates airway hyperresponsiveness.
- Common triggers of asthma exacerbations are preferentially mediated by neutrophilic airway inflammation. However, there exists no therapeutic approach that uniquely targets neutrophils in asthma.
- Targeting the activation state rather than the number of neutrophils may offer unique therapeutic approaches to improve asthma outcomes in patients with steroid-sensitive asthma.

INTRODUCTION

Asthma characterizes a complex syndrome manifested by airway obstruction, inflammation, and hyperresponsiveness. Contemporary thought suggests that patients with asthma exhibit marked heterogeneity in disease severity and in response to therapy. About 61% of adult patients with asthma exhibit allergen sensitivities or atopy, and 39% manifest little evidence of allergic disease.[1] Because the majority of patients with allergic disease and asthma demonstrate corticosteroid sensitivity, inhaled corticosteroids serves as a mainstay in asthma therapy. Despite this approach, at least 40% of patients are insensitive to inhaled corticosteroids and manifest a pathology that impugns neutrophils as important in asthma pathogenesis. To date, the mechanisms that regulate nonallergic asthma, traditionally known as intrinsic asthma, remain an unknown.

Disclosure Statement: Consultant/ad board, research grant, speaker: AstraZeneca, MedImmune. Consultant/ad board: Novartis. Research Grant: Theratrophix, Amgen, RIFM, Vertex, BMS, Gilead, Genentech, Sanofi, Regeneron, Speaker: Boston Scientific, Teva, Boehringer-Ingelheim.
Department of Medicine, Robert Wood Johnson Medical School, Rutgers Institute for Translational Medicine and Science, Rutgers, The State University of New Jersey, 89 French Street, Suite 4211, New Brunswick, NJ 08901, USA
E-mail address: rp856@rbhs.rutgers.edu

Immunol Allergy Clin N Am 38 (2018) 629–638
https://doi.org/10.1016/j.iac.2018.06.005
0889-8561/18/© 2018 Elsevier Inc. All rights reserved.
immunology.theclinics.com

Evidence suggests that neutrophil numbers in the bronchial wall or in sputum correlate with disease severity and are associated with asthma exacerbations.[2,3] Asthma exacerbations substantially contribute globally to morbidity, mortality, and health care costs.[4] Allergens, viruses, environmental tobacco smoke, and air pollution exposure commonly trigger exacerbations. Some, but not all, triggers respond to conventional therapy that includes oral glucocorticoids (GCs).[5,6] After allergen exposure, T-helper type 2 inflammation orchestrated by trafficking CD4-positive lymphocytes and eosinophils and by activation of mast cells evokes airway obstruction that reverses on treatment with GCs. Collectively, this cellular cascade defines a type 2 inflammatory response. Environmental tobacco smoke, ozone, or viruses, however, induce neutrophilic inflammation or directly modulate airway epithelial, smooth muscle, or neural cell function to evoke airway hyperresponsiveness and obstruction that is steroid insensitive.[4,7,8] Presumably, the direct effects of these triggers on airway structural cells may not induce typical type 2 responses but in part may be mediated by a T-helper type 1 (Th1) inflammatory response. In murine and human models of disease, studies suggest that non–type 2 responses (in the presence or absence of persistent type 2 inflammation) may be associated with severe airway obstruction that is, mediated by interferons (interferon-γ), T-helper type 17 , and nitric oxide production.[9] Typically, Th1 responses are steroid insensitive.[9] The lack of airway inflammatory cells or biomarkers in the presence of airway obstruction and airway hyperresponsiveness can also define pauci-immune or pauci-granulocytic asthma.[10] Characterization of novel therapeutic approaches targeting neutrophilic or pauci-immune asthma may have a profound impact on decreasing asthma exacerbations and improving asthma severity.

Using unbiased statistical approaches, cluster analyses organize patient data (blood samples, pulmonary function testing, and so forth) in a manner that demonstrates that some groups of patients are more similar than others according to mean vector connectivity (k-means algorithm).[10] Investigators have identified asthma clusters manifested by predominant neutrophilic inflammation, pauci-immune asthma, and steroid-insensitive disease.[10] Collectively, evidence suggests that some asthma exacerbations and specific asthma cohorts at baseline manifest predominantly neutrophilic phenotypes.

PATHOPHYSIOLOGY

A clinical syndrome manifested by limited numbers of eosinophils in the airways or peripheral circulation, nonatopy, rhinosinusitis with sleep disturbances, environmental tobacco smoke exposure, and gastroesophageal reflux disease characterize neutrophilic asthma.[11–13] Diagnostically, total sputum cell counts and neutrophil numbers are increased in comparison with those of healthy patients or patients with atopic asthma. Sputum neutrophil numbers, however, poorly correlate with methacholine responsiveness, whereas neutrophil numbers inversely correlate with pulmonary function.[13,14] In bronchial alveolar lavage and bronchial biopsies, numbers of neutrophils increase with more severe disease.[15–18] Evidence also suggests that sputum neutrophil numbers are associated with a progressive loss of lung function.[13,14] Because GCs increase neutrophil numbers in tissue and peripheral blood, the diagnosis can be complicated when patients are prescribed high-dose inhaled or oral steroids.[19] Given the efficacy of steroids to increase neutrophilia, this can serve as a biomarker of oral steroid adherence.

Investigators have also attempted to correlate neutrophil numbers in the sputum and peripheral blood in patients with asthma and comorbid diseases. Obesity, gastroesophageal reflux disease, and smoking are common comorbidities associated with difficult-to-manage asthma, steroid insensitivity, and non–type 2 responses. Unfortunately, whether neutrophil-mediated airway inflammation contributes to asthma disease severity associated with comorbidity remains controversial. In the Severe Asthma Research Program (SARP) and Unbiased Biomarkers in Prediction of Respiratory Disease Outcomes (UBIOPRED) cohorts, severe asthma was associated with gastroesophageal reflux disease but sputum neutrophilia was seen in only 1 cohort.[9] In obesity, sputum neutrophil numbers poorly correlated with asthma severity[9] and, although smoking increases neutrophils number in sputum from patients with asthma, cause and effect relationships among these covariates remain unknown.[9]

In many research studies, sputum neutrophils were used as a biomarker for neutrophil-mediated airway inflammation. Sputum analyses unfortunately require sophisticated training and limited availability hampers their clinical use. Discovery of other novel biomarkers to identify patients with neutrophilic asthma will foster precision approaches to improve therapy. Accordingly, levels of neutrophil-derived mediators (leukotriene B_4 [LTB_4], granulocyte-macrophage colony-stimulating factor, tumor necrosis factor-α [TNF-α], IL-17A, IL-8, elastase, or matrix metalloproteinase 9) are detectable in bronchial alveolar lavage fluid and plasma in patients with severe neutrophilic asthma.[2,16,18,20,21] Unlike eosinophilic asthma, systemic inflammation as measured by increased blood levels of IL-8, IL-6, C-reactive protein, and IL-17A was also reported in patients with severe neutrophilic asthma.[22] Although such blood levels hold promise, to date there exist no reliable serum biomarkers to diagnose neutrophilic asthma.

Conventional thought suggests that neutrophils primarily traffic to inflamed sites and then secrete granular enzymes, reactive oxygen species, and proteins to eliminate invading bacteria, fungal elements, and viruses. Undoubtedly, neutrophils play pivotal roles in innate immunity.[19] The 6- to 8-hour limited lifespan of the circulating neutrophil is consistent with an immune surveillance function.[23] Evidence also shows that some neutrophils survive much longer with lifespans of 3 to 5 days, especially in tissue.[17,24,25] Further, neutrophils can reenter the circulation via lymphatics and reverse migration through vascular endothelium.[26–28] Collectively, these observations suggest a more complex role of the neutrophil in modulating local inflammatory responses apart from host defense as shown in **Fig. 1**.

Given the differential lifespan of tissue and circulating neutrophils, these cells manifest unique functional phenotypes (**Table 1**). Mediated in part by granulocyte colony stimulating factor, granulocyte-macrophage colony-stimulating factor, interferon-γ, IL-13, LTB_4, and lipopolysaccharide,[17] tissue-based neutrophils have decreased apoptosis. Pertinent to severe asthma, neutrophil subsets can express FcγRIII (CD16) and FcϵRI and inhibit T-cell proliferation in a Mac-1- and H_2O_2-dependent manner.[29,30] Curiously, these neutrophils retain key innate effector cell functions, such as eliminating microbes.[31] Recruitment and retention of mucosal neutrophils, which are facilitated by T helper 17 cells (a subset of T helper lymphocytes releasing IL-17) induces secretion of IL-8 by airway epithelium.[32] Epithelial-induced secretion of IL-17 and IL-8 is also insensitive to GCs, a hallmark of severe neutrophilic asthma.[27] Neutrophils may transdifferentiate to express CD11a, CD11b, CD11c, HLA-DR, CD80, and CD86, acquiring an antigen-presenting cell phenotype (neutrophil/dendritic hybrid) in mice.[33] Whether such a transitional phenotype exists in severe asthma remains unknown. Collectively, current evidence suggests that neutrophils modulate adaptive responses and provide novel therapeutic targets for further exploration.

Repetitive injury of the airways from allergens, viruses, and toxicants in asthma evokes remodeling that increases matrix deposition, airway smooth muscle mass,

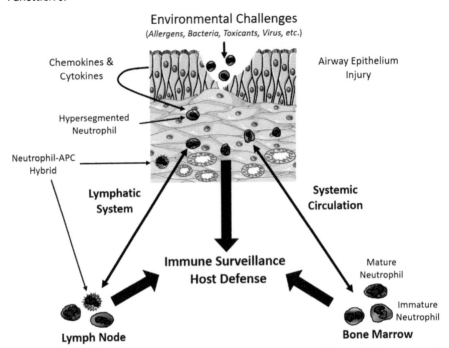

Fig. 1. Neutrophil subsets mediate immune surveillance and host defense. Evidence suggests that neutrophil subsets may mediate differential effects on immune surveillance and microbial killing. A variety of epithelial insults (ozone, bacteria, and viruses) induce secretion of chemokines and cytokines that promote neutrophil trafficking. Most circulating neutrophils are a mature phenotype (neu-2). On injury other phenotypes appear, namely neu-1, the immature or band neutrophil, and neu-3, the hypersegmented neutrophil. During asthma exacerbations, the presence of chemokines and cytokines (IL-8, IL-17A, and so forth) prolongs the lifespan of the neutrophil and modulates T-helper type 2 and innate immune responses. The prolonged lifespan also enables neutrophils to migrate from tissue to the systemic circulation or to lymph nodes to modulate adaptive immune responses. (*Adapted from* Panettieri RA. Neutrophilic and pauciimmune phenotypes in severe asthma. Immunol Allergy Clin North Am 2016;36(3):572; with permission.)

Table 1
Neutrophil subsets manifest specific phenotypes

Neutrophil Attributes	Immature	Mature	Hypersegmented
Nuclei morphology	Band	Segmented	Multilobed
L-selectin (CD62 L)[a]	+	+	−
FcγRIII (CD16)[a]	−	+	+
T-cell suppression	−	−	+
Lifespan	Hours	Hours	Days
Neutrophil-APC hybrid	−	−	+
Activated[b]	−	−	+
Microbial killing	−	+	+

Abbreviation: APC, antigen-presenting cell.
 [a] Cell surface expression.
 [b] Activated: Capable of endocytosis, neutrophil extracellular net formation, and MPO and matrix metalloproteinase production.
From Panettieri RA. Neutrophilic and pauciimmune phenotypes in severe asthma. Immunol Allergy Clin North Am 2016;36(3):573; with permission.

mucus gland hypertrophy, and angiogenesis.[4,7,8] The physiologic consequences of remodeling events in the pathogenesis of irreversible airway obstruction remains unclear.[8] Activated neutrophils secrete transforming growth factor-β, matrix metalloproteinase 9, elastase, and myeloperoxidase.[14] In bronchial alveolar lavage, matrix metalloproteinase 9 levels correlate with neutrophil counts in asthma.[34] Taken together, neutrophils may play a role in promoting airway remodeling, but this notion remains controversial.

Are There Targeted Therapies for Neutrophilic Asthma?

There currently exist no therapies approved by the US Food and Drug Administration for neutrophilic asthma. Clinicians typically prescribe combined therapies of inhaled GCs and long-acting bronchodilators as a cornerstone of medical management. Disappointingly, this approach often fails to improve pulmonary function or functional status in patients with neutrophilic asthma.[35] The presence of submucosal or airway neutrophils suggests that the trafficking or activation state of the neutrophil may serve as a therapeutic target. Strategies to alter neutrophil function can include blockade of chemokine receptors (CXCR2 antagonists); inhibition of the effects of TNF-α, IL-6, or IL-17; kinase inhibition (p38MAPK, PI3K-d/g, JAK, or PDE4); or macrolides. However, such approaches remain investigational.

Chemokines (CXCL1 [GRO-a], CXCL5 [ENA- 78], CXCL8 [IL-8], and LTB$_4$) modulate neutrophil migration by activating G-protein–coupled receptors CXCR2 or, in the case of LTB$_4$, the LTB$_4$ receptor 2.[19] Accordingly, blockade of these receptors would decrease neutrophil trafficking and in turn inflammatory responses. CXCR2 inhibition significantly decreased sputum neutrophils, but only modestly decreased mild exacerbations and had no effect on pulmonary function in patients with chronic obstructive pulmonary disease.[36] Significant decreases in circulating neutrophils induced by CXCR2 blockade but had little effect on pulmonary function or functional status in patients with severe asthma.[37] Further, blockade of 5-lipoxygenase that decreases LTB$_4$ and leukotriene D4 levels offers therapeutic benefit in asthma associated with aspirin sensitivity and nasal polyps; the relative contribution of LTB$_4$ and leukotriene D4 in improving patient outcomes in neutrophilic asthma remains unclear. Despite the targeting inhibition of neutrophil chemotaxis, the lack of clinical improvements and the possibility for neutropenia with immunosuppression limit the therapeutic value of this target in severe asthma.

Neutrophilic asthma is associated with increased levels of TNF-α, IL-6, or IL-17 in the blood or sputum of patients.[14,19] Investigators have posited that binding free circulating cytokines or inhibition of their cognate receptor may improve clinical outcomes. Inhibiting the actions of TNF-α or IL-17 with monoclonal antibodies provided marginal therapeutic advantages in severe asthma.[38–40] Whether such agents would be effective in neutrophilic asthma remains unclear because the clinical trials were not designed to assess efficacy in this cohort.

Extracellular signals via activation of receptors stimulate intracellular kinases (p38MAPK, JNK, PI3K-δ/γ, and JAK) and phosphodiesterases (PDEs) that modulate cell proliferation, chemokine and cytokine production, apoptosis, and steroid sensitivity. Each of these kinases or PDEs selectively modulates neutrophil secretion, diapedesis, and apoptosis.[14,19] Despite intracellular kinase inhibitors being developed for chronic obstructive pulmonary disease, such agents may also have usefulness in neutrophilic asthma.[35] Interestingly, p38MAPK and JNK1 activation also phosphorylates the GC receptor that inhibits its translocation into the nucleus, which is necessary to mediate GCs' antiinflammatory effects.[35] Using cell culture models, blockade of p38MAPK or JNK1 reverses steroid insensitivity.[35] Whether such mechanisms are physiologically relevant in neutrophilic asthma remains unknown. Unfortunately, given the ubiquitous expression of intracellular kinases, their inhibition may evoke undesirable adverse effects that include immunosuppression or malignancy.

In some cell types, cAMP or cGMP work intracellularly as antiinflammatory signaling molecules; blockade of PDEs, which increase cAMP and cGMP levels, would amplify these antiinflammatory responses.[35] PDEs decrease cAMP or cGMP levels and diminishes activation of protein kinase A or G, respectively. In circulating immunocytes, PDE4 is the dominant isoform. Roflumilast, a PDE4 inhibitor, improved neutrophil-mediated airway inflammation and decreased exacerbations[41] in chronic obstructive pulmonary disease; whether such effects would have therapeutic benefit in neutrophilic asthma remains unknown.

Macrolide antibiotics used to treat chronic indolent infections with atypical bacteria (*Mycoplasma pneumonia* or *Chlamydia pneumonia*) improved patient-reported outcomes in patients with severe asthma.[42,43] The role of chronic infection in the pathogenesis of severe asthma remains controversial. Arguably, macrolide antibiotics can also act as antiinflammatory agents with a mechanism of action disparate from any antiinfective activity. Macrolides inhibit nuclear factor-kB activation and secretion of CXCL8 and promote phagocytosis.[44,45] In severe asthma, azithromycin reduced sputum neutrophil counts and CXCL8 levels with improved patient-reported outcomes in patients with neutrophilic inflammation.[46,47] Taken together, the current evidence suggests that macrolide antibiotics may have value in neutrophilic asthma; the low risk of complications justifies a 6-month clinical trial in some patients prone to exacerbations.

The therapeutic benefit of combined long-acting beta agonists and anticholinergic agents is well-established in chronic obstructive pulmonary disease. Further, the addition of antimuscarinic agents in the treatment of severe asthma is a therapy approved by the US Food and Drug Administration.[35] Whether such approaches would have preferential effects in neutrophilic asthma as compared with those in eosinophilic asthma remains unclear. Few studies have focused on therapeutic approaches of bronchial thermoplasty in neutrophilic asthma. Bronchial thermoplasty delivers thermal energy to the airway in a manner that ultimately remodels the airway epithelium and decreases airway smooth muscle mass in the proximal airways.[48] The therapeutic improvement in exacerbations did not extinguish over 5 years of observation.[49] Other studies now show that bronchial thermoplasty also modulates mucosal inflammatory responses and collagen deposition.[50–52] Because patients who undergo bronchial thermoplasty are poor candidates for T-helper type 2 or IgE monoclonal antibody therapies or have failed such approaches, bronchial thermoplasty may become the treatment of choice for neutrophilic severe asthma. Further studies, however, are needed to definitively show efficacy in these cohorts.

Neutrophilic Asthma: Many Unanswered Questions

Despite considerable efforts to therapeutically target neutrophilic asthma, few approaches have improved patient outcomes.[14,19,35] Health care providers, when faced with a patient refractory to treatment, typically prescribe oral GCs. Unfortunately, oral GCs promote neutrophil survival and increase neutrophil numbers, providing a diagnostic dilemma. Given the failure of current approaches to improve outcomes in neutrophilic asthma, a fresh approach is needed. Perhaps the global inhibition of neutrophils in the circulation or airways may not be an effective therapeutic target. Compelling evidence suggests that some subsets of neutrophils provide a negative homeostatic function to inhibit inflammation, whereas others may amplify antigen presentation and T-helper type 2 inflammation.[14,19] A greater understanding of the heterogeneity of neutrophil responses and subsets may improve awareness that global targeting of neutrophil activation or trafficking will be uninformative. Improved phenotyping of patients with neutrophilic asthma will identify specific neutrophil endotypes that will predict therapeutic responses.

SUMMARY AND FUTURE CONSIDERATIONS

Asthma represents as a complex syndrome defined in part by reversible airway obstruction and inflammation. Although our understanding of eosinophil- and type 2-mediated inflammation in asthma has improved, our knowledge regarding neutrophilic disease remains rudimentary. Because the neutrophil may play an important role in mediating the asthma diathesis in some cohorts, we need novel therapeutic targets to modulate neutrophil activation or migration. Although drugs are early in development, the proposed targets may not uniformly offer therapeutic efficacy. Given the heterogeneity among neutrophil subsets, research paradigms should consider that global inhibition of neutrophil activation and migration may be inappropriate and may induced unwanted adverse effects. Improved characterization of neutrophil subsets and the development of accurate biomarkers to predict therapeutic responses may improve clinical outcomes. Because neutrophilic and pauci-granulocytic asthma are steroid insensitive, our current approaches of using oral steroids in refractory asthma patients with neutrophil inflammation may offer little therapeutic benefit while increasing adverse effects.

REFERENCES

1. Knudsen TB, Thomsen SF, Nolte H, et al. A population-based clinical study of allergic and non-allergic asthma. J Asthma 2009;1:91–4.
2. Jatakanon A, Uasuf C, Maziak W, et al. Neutrophilic inflammation in severe persistent asthma. Am J Respir Crit Care Med 1999;(5 Pt 1):1532–9.
3. Norzila MZ, Fakes K, Henry RL, et al. Interleukin-8 secretion and neutrophil recruitment accompanies induced sputum eosinophil activation in children with acute asthma. Am J Respir Crit Care Med 2000;(3 Pt 1):769–74.
4. Koziol-White CJ, Panettieri RA Jr. Airway smooth muscle and immunomodulation in acute exacerbations of airway disease. Immunol Rev 2011;242(1):178–85.
5. Athens JW, Haab OP, Raab SO, et al. Leukokinetic studies. IV. The total blood, circulating and marginal granulocyte pools and the granulocyte turnover rate in normal subjects. J Clin Invest 1961;989–95.
6. Hetherington SV, Quie PG. Human polymorphonuclear leukocytes of the bone marrow, circulation, and marginated pool: function and granule protein content. Am J Hematol 1985;235–46.
7. Damera G, Panettieri RA Jr. Does airway smooth muscle express an inflammatory phenotype in asthma? Br J Pharmacol 2011;1:68–80.
8. Damera G, Panettieri RA. Irreversible airway obstruction in asthma: what we lose, we lose early. Allergy Asthma Proc 2014;2:111–8.
9. Ray A, Kolls JK. Neutrophilic inflammation in asthma and association with disease severity. Trends Immunol 2017;12:942–54.
10. Chung KF. Defining phenotypes in asthma: a step towards personalized medicine. Drugs 2014;7:719–28.
11. Baines KJ, Simpson JL, Wood LG, et al. Systemic upregulation of neutrophil alpha-defensins and serine proteases in neutrophilic asthma. Thorax 2011;11:942–7.

12. Douwes J, Gibson P, Pekkanen J, et al. Non-eosinophilic asthma: importance and possible mechanisms. Thorax 2002;7:643–8.
13. Simpson JL, Baines KJ, Ryan N, et al. Neutrophilic asthma is characterised by increased rhinosinusitis with sleep disturbance and GERD. Asian Pac J Allergy Immunol 2014;1:66–74.
14. Shaw DE, Berry MA, Hargadon B, et al. Association between neutrophilic airway inflammation and airflow limitation in adults with asthma. Chest 2007;6:1871–5.
15. Louis R, Lau LC, Bron AO, et al. The relationship between airways inflammation and asthma severity. Am J Respir Crit Care Med 2000;1:9–16.
16. Teran LM, Campos MG, Begishvilli BT, et al. Identification of neutrophil chemotactic factors in bronchoalveolar lavage fluid of asthmatic patients. Clin Exp Allergy 1997;4:396–405.
17. Uddin M, Nong G, Ward J, et al. Prosurvival activity for airway neutrophils in severe asthma. Thorax 2010;8:684–9.
18. Wenzel SE, Szefler SJ, Leung DY, et al. Bronchoscopic evaluation of severe asthma. Persistent inflammation associated with high dose glucocorticoids. Am J Respir Crit Care Med 1997;(3 Pt 1):737–43.
19. Bruijnzeel PL, Uddin M, Koenderman L. Targeting neutrophilic inflammation in severe neutrophilic asthma: can we target the disease-relevant neutrophil phenotype? J Leukoc Biol 2015;4:549–56.
20. Simpson JL, Grissell TV, Douwes J, et al. Innate immune activation in neutrophilic asthma and bronchiectasis. Thorax 2007;3:211–8.
21. Uddin M, Lau LC, Seumois G, et al. EGF-induced bronchial epithelial cells drive neutrophil chemotactic and anti-apoptotic activity in asthma. PLoS One 2013;9: e72502.
22. Wood LG, Baines KJ, Fu J, et al. The neutrophilic inflammatory phenotype is associated with systemic inflammation in asthma. Chest 2012;1:86–93.
23. Shi J, Gilbert GE, Kokubo Y, et al. Role of the liver in regulating numbers of circulating neutrophils. Blood 2001;4:1226–30.
24. Dancey JT, Deubelbeiss KA, Harker LA, et al. Neutrophil kinetics in man. J Clin Invest 1976;3:705–15.
25. Pillay J, Kamp VM, van Hoffen E, et al. A subset of neutrophils in human systemic inflammation inhibits T cell responses through Mac-1. J Clin Invest 2012;1: 327–36.
26. Buckley CD, Ross EA, McGettrick HM, et al. Identification of a phenotypically and functionally distinct population of long-lived neutrophils in a model of reverse endothelial migration. J Leukoc Biol 2006;2:303–11.
27. Bullens DM, Truyen E, Coteur L, et al. IL-17 mRNA in sputum of asthmatic patients: linking T cell driven inflammation and granulocytic influx? Respir Res 2006;7:135.
28. Woodfin A, Voisin MB, Beyrau M, et al. The junctional adhesion molecule JAM-C regulates polarized transendothelial migration of neutrophils in vivo. Nat Immunol 2011;8:761–9.
29. Gounni AS, Lamkhioued B, Koussih L, et al. Human neutrophils express the high-affinity receptor for immunoglobulin E (Fc epsilon RI): role in asthma. FASEB J 2001;6:940–9.
30. Maletto BA, Ropolo AS, Alignani DO, et al. Presence of neutrophil-bearing antigen in lymphoid organs of immune mice. Blood 2006;9:3094–102.
31. Geng S, Matsushima H, Okamoto T, et al. Emergence, origin, and function of neutrophil-dendritic cell hybrids in experimentally induced inflammatory lesions in mice. Blood 2013;10:1690–700.

32. Cosmi L, Annunziato F, Galli MIG, et al. CRTH2 is the most reliable marker for the detection of circulating human type 2 Th and type 2 T cytotoxic cells in health and disease. Eur J Immunol 2000;10:2972–9.

33. Matsushima H, Geng S, Lu R, et al. Neutrophil differentiation into a unique hybrid population exhibiting dual phenotype and functionality of neutrophils and dendritic cells. Blood 2013;10:1677–89.

34. Banerjee A, Damera G, Bhandare R, et al. Vitamin D and glucocorticoids differentially modulate chemokine expression in human airway smooth muscle cells. Br J Pharmacol 2008;1:84–92.

35. Barnes PJ. Therapeutic approaches to asthma-chronic obstructive pulmonary disease overlap syndromes. J Allergy Clin Immunol 2015;3:531–45.

36. Magnussen H, Watz H, Sauer M, et al. Safety and efficacy of SCH527123, a novel CXCR2 antagonist, in patients with COPD. Eur Respir J 2010;38S:1097–103.

37. Nair P, Gaga M, Zervas E, et al. Safety and efficacy of a CXCR2 antagonist in patients with severe asthma and sputum neutrophils: a randomized, placebo-controlled clinical trial. Clin Exp Allergy 2012;7:1097–103.

38. Al-Ramli W, Prefontaine D, Chouiali F, et al. T(H)17-associated cytokines (IL-17A and IL-17F) in severe asthma. J Allergy Clin Immunol 2009;5:1185–7.

39. Chesne J, Braza F, Mahay G, et al. IL-17 in severe asthma. Where do we stand? Am J Respir Crit Care Med 2014;10:1094–101.

40. Wenzel SE, Barnes PJ, Bleecker ER, et al. A randomized, double-blind, placebo-controlled study of tumor necrosis factor-alpha blockade in severe persistent asthma. Am J Respir Crit Care Med 2009;7:549–58.

41. Calverley PM, Rabe KF, Goehring UM, et al. M & groups, M.s. Roflumilast in symptomatic chronic obstructive pulmonary disease: two randomised clinical trials. Lancet 2009;9691:685–94.

42. Kraft M, Cassell GH, Pak J, et al. Mycoplasma pneumoniae and Chlamydia pneumoniae in asthma: effect of clarithromycin. Chest 2002;6:1782–8.

43. Sutherland ER, King TS, Icitovic N, et al, National Heart, Lung & Blood Institute's Asthma Clinical Research, Network. A trial of clarithromycin for the treatment of suboptimally controlled asthma. J Allergy Clin Immunol 2010;4:747–53.

44. Hodge S, Hodge G, Brozyna S, et al. Azithromycin increases phagocytosis of apoptotic bronchial epithelial cells by alveolar macrophages. Eur Respir J 2006;3:486–95.

45. Kobayashi Y, Wada H, Rossios C, et al. A novel macrolide solithromycin exerts superior anti-inflammatory effect via NF-kappaB inhibition. J Pharmacol Exp Ther 2013;1:76–84.

46. Brusselle GG, Vanderstichele C, Jordens P, et al. Azithromycin for prevention of exacerbations in severe asthma (AZISAST): a multicentre randomised double-blind placebo-controlled trial. Thorax 2013;4:322–9.

47. Simpson JL, Powell H, Boyle MJ, et al. Clarithromycin targets neutrophilic airway inflammation in refractory asthma. Am J Respir Crit Care Med 2008;2:148–55.

48. Castro M, Rubin AS, Laviolette M, et al. Effectiveness and safety of bronchial thermoplasty in the treatment of severe asthma: a multicenter, randomized, double-blind, sham-controlled clinical trial. Am J Respir Crit Care Med 2010;2:116–24.

49. Wechsler ME, Laviolette M, Rubin AS, et al, Asthma Intervention Research 2 Trial Study, Group. Bronchial thermoplasty: long-term safety and effectiveness in patients with severe persistent asthma. J Allergy Clin Immunol 2013;6:1295–302.

50. Chakir J, Haj-Salem I, Gras D, et al. Effects of bronchial thermoplasty on airway smooth muscle and collagen deposition in asthma. Ann Am Thorac Soc 2015; 12(11):1612–8.

51. Denner DR, Doeing DC, Hogarth DK, et al. Airway inflammation after bronchial thermoplasty for severe asthma. Ann Am Thorac Soc 2015;9:1302–9.

52. Panettieri RA Jr. Bronchial thermoplasty: targeting structural cells in severe persistent asthma. Ann Am Thorac Soc 2015;11:1593–4.

Airway Eosinophilopoietic and Autoimmune Mechanisms of Eosinophilia in Severe Asthma

Anurag Bhalla, MD[1], Manali Mukherjee, PhD[1],
Parameswaran Nair, MD, PhD, FRCP, FRCPC*

KEYWORDS

- Severe asthma • Sputum eosinophils • IL-5 • In situ eosinophilopoiesis
- Autoantibodies • Steroid insensitivity

KEY POINTS

- Local eosinophilopoietic processes may play a significant role in perpetuating eosinophilic inflammation in the lungs in severe asthma.
- Innate lymphoid cell group 2 may also be a key mediator in maintaining airway eosinophilia in patients with severe asthma.
- Persistent airway eosinophilia may be a reflection of steroid insensitivity.
- Persistent luminal eosinophilic activity, together with recurrent airway infections, may lead to airway autoimmune responses that may further contribute to steroid insensitivity.
- Clinical responses to antiinterleukin-5 therapies may depend on their dosing and routes of administration, mechanisms of action, and the autoimmune responses in the airway.

INTRODUCTION

More than a century ago, Paul Ehrlich stained eosinophils in blood smears (1879). Decades later, eosinophils were stained in the sputum of an asthmatic.[1,2] The study by Harry Morrow Brown[2] further established the therapeutic effect of corticosteroid

Disclosure Statement: P. Nair is supported by the Frederick E. Hargreave Teva Innovation Chair in Airway Diseases. In the past 2 years, he has received consultancy and lecture fees from Astra-Zeneca, Sanofi, Teva, Novartis, Theravance, Knopp, Merck, GlaxoSmithKline, and Roche; research support from GlaxoSmithKline, AstraZeneca, and Novartis; and his institution has received research support from Roche, Teva, Sanofi, Boehringer Ingelheim, AstraZeneca, and Novartis. M. Mukherjee and A. Bhalla do not have any conflicts to declare.
Division of Respirology, Firestone Institute for Respiratory Health, St Joseph's Healthcare, McMaster University, 50 Charlton Avenue East, Hamilton, Ontario L8N 4A6, Canada
[1] Equal contributions.
* Corresponding author.
E-mail address: parames@mcmaster.ca

Immunol Allergy Clin N Am 38 (2018) 639–654
https://doi.org/10.1016/j.iac.2018.06.003
immunology.theclinics.com

treatment (prednisolone) in ameliorating asthma symptoms and related it to the presence of airway (sputum) eosinophils. Unanimously considered to be a heterogeneous disease, asthma is defined by the presence of reversible airflow obstruction, airway hyperresponsiveness, and/or airway inflammation,[3] in which 40% of patients exhibit eosinophil-driven pathobiology.[3,4] Corticosteroids have remained the mainstay treatment of asthma and reduction in eosinophils has remained the unequivocal predictor of steroid response.[3,5]

The severity of asthma is evaluated by increased use of corticosteroids (inhaled and/or oral) and the inability to achieve optimal asthma control (ie, relief of symptoms and reduction in exacerbations) despite daily use.[6,7] Typically, asthmatics are prednisone-dependent, have difficult to control symptoms, and present with persistent airway eosinophilia,[8] often not reflected in the peripheral circulation.[9] This review article focuses on the novel mechanisms involved in persistent eosinophilia in airways, including in situ eosinophilopoiesis, and on steroid insensitivity, leading to persistent eosinophilia with contributing airway infections and autoimmune responses.

IMMUNOBIOLOGY OF EOSINOPHILS IN ASTHMA

Past decades of intense research into the role of eosinophils in pathologic asthma has revealed the versatility of these granulocytes, which were originally thought to be end-effector cells for host defense against helminth infection.[10,11] With respect to asthma, eosinophils have been implicated as mediators of both innate and adaptive immunity.[10] Direct and indirect evidences have shown eosinophils to be involved in T-cell proliferation, activation, including T helper (Th) cells with type 1 (Th1) or type 2 (Th2) polarization, as well as in antigen presentation in response to certain bacterial, viral, and parasitic infections.[12] In addition to eosinophil-derived inflammatory mediators, cytokines,[13] the granule proteins released by activated eosinophils, have established role in asthma pathology capable of inducing tissue damage, activating mucosal mast cell and basophil degranulation, increasing smooth muscle reactivity, and secreting additional immune mediators.[11,14] The release of cytotoxic cationic granular proteins is primarily regulated by various degrees of degranulation machineries, namely exocytosis, cytolysis, piecemeal degranulation,[14,15] and the recently described eosinophil-derived extracellular DNA traps (EETs).[16] In fact, increased eosinophil peroxidase (EPX) and free eosinophil granules, which are known markers of heightened airway eosinophil activity, are associated with indices of asthma severity.[17,18]

CAUSES OF PERSISTENT AIRWAY EOSINOPHILIA

It is important to briefly mention the conventionally accepted pathways that lead to genesis of eosinophilia before delving into the alternative pathways. Eosinophilopoiesis is a term that encompasses all factors that govern the initial eosinophil lineage commitment, differentiation, and maturation in bone marrow, followed by the proliferation, survival, and migration into the peripheral tissues via circulation.[19] Eosinophilopoietic mechanisms and recruitment of eosinophils into the lung tissue are crucial for orchestrating the eosinophilic airway inflammation central to asthma pathobiology; they have been reviewed extensively[20] (Fig. 1). Under inflammatory conditions, eosinophils are trafficked to the lung in response to Th2 cytokines (ie, interleukin [IL]-4, IL-5, and IL-13),[21] aided by upregulation of adhesion molecules[22] and chemokine signaling (CCL5, eotaxins 1, 2, and 3).[23,24] IL-5 is the most critical eosinophilopoietic cytokine (extensively reviewed elsewhere[25,26]) and plays a pivotal role in eosinophilopoiesis and as end-stage effector functions (see Fig. 1).

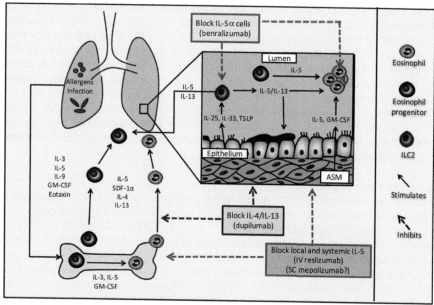

Fig. 1. Local and systemic factors contributing to airway eosinophilia and therapeutic strategies to block them. ASM, airway smooth muscle; GM-CSF, granulocyte-macrophage colony-stimulating factor; IL, interleukin; IV, intravenous; SDF, stromal derived factor; TSLP, thymic stromal lymphopoietin. Question mark indicates unconfirmed status of whether the drug at 100 mg dosage, administered subcutaneously, reduces local IL5.

In Situ Eosinophilopoiesis

It is well-established that eosinophilopoiesis is not limited to the bone marrow. Indeed, $CD34^+$ cells extracted from human nasal polyp or explant tissue readily undergo IL-5–driven differentiation to form mature eosinophils in vitro.[27,28] Increased numbers of eosinophil progenitors (EoPs) have been reported in the sera of atopic patients[29] and bronchial mucosa of mild asthmatics post an allergen challenge.[30] Compared with mild asthmatics, a significantly greater number of $CD34^+$ hematopoietic cells (HPCs), mature eosinophils and EoPs ($CD34^+45^+$IL-5 [receptor] $R\alpha^+$) were enumerated in sputum of severe asthmatics. Furthermore, using IL-5–supplemented 14-day culture of methylcellulose colony assays, blood EoPs from severe asthmatics demonstrated greater clonogenic potential than that from mild asthmatics, as measured by growth of eosinophil-basophil–colony-forming units (Eo/B-CFUs).[31] The persistence of sputum EoPs in severe asthmatics despite treatment with an anti–IL-5 monoclonal antibody (mAb) was associated with persistent sputum eosinophils and a lower prednisone-sparing effect.[31] These observations, coupled with the lack of efficacy of the CCR3 antagonist (receptor for eotaxins) in suppressing circulating and airway eosinophils in moderate-to-severe asthmatics,[32] suggests that in situ eosinophilopoiesis as a predominant mechanisms contributes to the persistence of airway eosinophilia in addition to the chemokine (eg, eotaxin 2 or 3)-dependent eosinophil recruitment from peripheral blood. Finally, in situ eosinophilopoiesis is not exclusively limited to IL-5 and may be driven by several factors (see later discussion).

T helper type 2 cytokines: interleukin-4 and interleukin-13

Conventionally, IL-4 is known to promote differentiation of Th2 cells and isotype class switching to immunoglobulin (Ig)E, whereas IL-13 induces IgE secretion[33] and is predominately associated with goblet cell hyperplasia, airway smooth muscle (ASM) cell hypertrophy, and subepithelial fibrosis.[34] Type I IL-4 Rα and IL-4Rγc are selectively activated by IL-4, whereas type II IL-4Rα and IL-13Rα1 are activated by both IL-4 and IL-13.[33] The alternative (IL-13Rα2) is a decoy receptor.[35] Both IL-13 and IL-4 induce eotaxins 1, 2, and 3 release from diverse cellular sources, which are potent eosinophil chemoattractants.[24] Again, stromal cell-derived factor (SDF)-1α is a potent progenitor cell chemoattractant and acts via G-protein coupled receptor, CXCR4.[36] IL-4 and IL-13 are responsible for priming SDF-1α–stimulated migration of the HPCs.[37] In contrast, IL-4 and IL-13 do not prime SDF-1α–directed migration of EoPs or mature eosinophils; nonetheless, they do prime the migration of mature eosinophils to eotaxins.

T helper cell type 2 alarmins

Epithelial-derived alarmins, such as thymic stromal lymphopoietin (TSLP), IL-33, and IL-25, are released on extraneous stimuli and have established roles in promoting the submucosal Th2 cascade in asthma.[38,39] Both IL-33[40] and TSLP[41,42] expression are increased in airways of asthmatics and correlate with disease severity. In particular, after an allergen challenge, a significant increase in sputum CD34$^+$ HPCs and EoPs have been observed, with increased expression of TSLP receptor components (CD127) and IL-33R (ST2). Moreover, overnight incubation of HPCs with TSLP and IL-33 independently enhanced migration of HPC to CXCL12, a potent progenitor cell chemoattractant, an effect that was attenuated with neutralizing antibodies for both TSLP and IL-33.[43] Moreover, using an IL-13Rα1 antibody but not IL-4Rα, there was inhibition of the priming effect of TSLP and IL-33 to CXCL12-stimulated migration of HPCs, thereby suggesting downstream role of IL-13 in lung homing of progentiors.[44] Isolated CD34$^+$ cells stimulated with TSLP in combination with IL-5 also increased expression of GATA-2 and C/EBPα, key transcriptional factors involved in eosinophil development.[43] The study concluded that in an IL-5–rich environment, TSLP promotes progenitor recruitment, eosinophilic lineage commitment, and in situ eosinophilopoiesis. More recently, the immediate downstream effector function of the alarmins has been associated with activation of the newly described innate lymphoid cells (ILCs) that express the receptors for these alarmins.

Lung-resident innate lymphoid cells group 2

ILCs, derived from common lymphoid progenitors in bone marrow, lack both B-cell and T-cell receptors, and play a diverse role in inflammation and tissue remodeling.[45] Retinoid-related orphan receptor (ROR)α and GATA-3 are key transcription factors involved in polarizing the ILCs to group 2 (ILC2) differentiation and function. Specifically, ILC2s reside in lung tissue (in response to the chemoattractant effects mediated through the CRTH2 receptor signaling) and have been found to be a potent source of type-2 cytokines.[46] As previously mentioned, ILC2s express receptors for IL-25 and IL-33; therefore, they have been shown to play a critical role in initiating type 2 responses in the airways,[47] with IL-33 being more potent than IL-25 in vitro.[48] In subjects with prednisone-dependent severe eosinophilic asthma, ILC2s were significantly increased in both circulation (blood) and sputum. However, in subjects with persistent airway eosinophilia ($\geq$3% eosinophils) and normal blood eosinophils (<300 cells/μL), there was an increase in "IL-5$^+$IL-13$^+$ILC2" in sputum compared with circulation. In addition, though the CD4$^+$ lymphocyte population was enumerated to be greater than the ILC2s in the airways, the latter was seen to be the predominant source of type 2 cytokines, IL-5, and IL-13.[49] In summary, in severe asthmatics, IL-13 primes progenitor cell migration by SDF-1α, hence promoting EoPs homing into the lung,[37] whereas persistent IL-5 production by the lung-resident ILC2s provide a signal for maturation of EoPs in situ. Taken together, these indicate that ILC2s may be responsible for maintaining persistent airway eosinophilia.[49]

Airway structural cells: epithelial cells and airway smooth muscle

Airway epithelial cells provide a regulated interface between the host and the environment, and are often the first line of defense. Epithelial cells express many pattern recognition receptors, including toll-like receptors, NOD-like receptors, C-type lectins, and protease-activated receptors.[50] On activation from environmental stimuli (allergens, pollutants, viruses, or bacteria), epithelial cells are capable of inducing type 2 eosinophilic inflammatory events via release of alarmins (see previous discussion). Additionally, epigenetic changes in the bronchial epithelium are responsible for production of IL-33.[51,52] In vitro bronchial epithelial cell supernatant BECSN cocultures with nonadherent mononuclear cells containing an enriched population of CD34+ HPCs stimulated clonogenic expansion of eosinophilic progenitors. This expansion was significantly increased with coadministration of IL-5. Eo/B-CFUs were significantly greater in cocultures of BECSN from severe asthmatics compared with mild asthmatics. This increase was attenuated in presence of TSLP-blocking antibodies but not IL-5Rα or ST-2–blocking (against IL-33) antibodies.[43]

Traditionally, ASM was thought to be responsible for bronchomotor tone under neurohormonal and inflammatory influences.[53] However, recent evidence suggests that ASM may play a role in maintaining airway inflammation by secreting a host of chemokines and cytokines.[54] ASMs derived from nonasthmatics, in the presence of stimulating cytokines (tumor necrosis factor-α, interferon-γ, and IL-1β), produced granulocyte-macrophage colony-stimulating factor (GM-CSF), CCL5, IL-5, IL-8, and eotaxin in vitro. Moreover, HPCs co-cultured with stimulated ASMs demonstrated a clonogenic response (measured as presence of Eo/B-CFUs). In presence of neutralizing antibodies to IL-5 and GM-CSF, this eosinophilopoietic response was attenuated.[55] Thus, ASM cells have the ability to direct eosinophil differentiation and maturation from progenitor cells, which could contribute to persistent eosinophilia.

Glucocorticosteroid Subsensitivity

Glucocorticosteroid (GCS) treatment is primarily targeted toward suppressing the eosinophilic component. The mechanisms of action of GCSs have been extensively reviewed.[56] "Lower than expected GCS response" is termed steroid subsensitivity and is considered to be among the primary mechanisms that contribute to persistent airway eosinophilia. The term is collective and encompasses steroid-resistant and steroid-insensitive asthmatics. Of current interest are patients who are steroid insensitive; that is, patients who remain poorly controlled despite maximal treatment (generally daily maintenance prednisone) or experience loss of asthma control during dose reduction or discontinuation. The heterogeneity in the underlying mechanisms leading to persistent eosinophilia despite GCS therapy is extensively studied.[56,57] Genetic factors and consequent aberrations in receptor biology are outside the scope of this discussion and have been extensively reviewed.[56] The underlying mechanisms leading to steroid insensitivity and associated persistent airway eosinophilia can be construed to be a part of disease progression, unlike that of patients who are steroid-unresponsive or steroid-resistant (ie, those who do not respond to GCSs, with no clinically relevant improvement in lung function or reduction in eosinophils following 14 days of prednisone, 40 mg/d). See later discussion of 2 novel mechanisms resulting from chronic inflammation that could contribute to steroid insensitivity (**Fig. 2**).

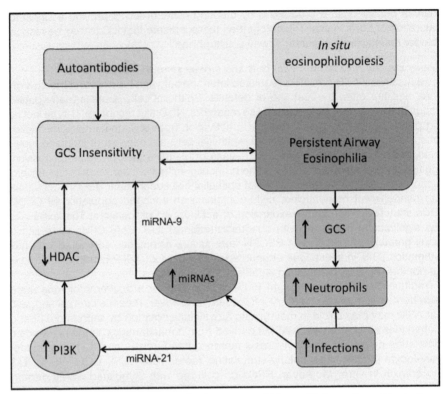

Fig. 2. Schematic of pathways contributing to steroid insensitivity and persistent airway eosinophilia. GCS, glucocorticosteroid; HDAC, histone deacetylase; miRNA, micro-RNA; PI3K, phosphoinositide 3-kinase.

Autoimmune responses following chronic inflammation

Eosinophils exert their toxic effect by primary lysis and release of free eosinophilic granules (containing tissue-toxic cationic proteins) and danger-associated molecular patterns.[17] Over time, eosinophilic inflammation leads to accumulation of self-antigens such as EPX, thereby fostering a microenvironment that could potentially lead to breach of immune tolerance. Indeed, patients with severe eosinophilic asthma have detectable IgG antibodies against EPX and other autologous cellular components, such as dsDNA, histones, and so forth (collectively termed antinuclear antibodies [ANAs]) in the sputum. These antibodies are present in much lower titers in serum, suggesting the presence of in situ mechanisms in the airway that promote autoantibody generation. Moreover, airway autoantibodies were associated with clinical markers of airway eosinophilic degranulation (sputum EPX and free eosinophil granules), as well as the ex vivo phenomenon of (EETs) and associated dsDNA release. Ex vivo formation of EETs on stimulation with sputum autoantibodies could not be suppressed by dexamethasone, which further supported the significant association between anti-EPX IgG and the dose of maintenance prednisone.[58] Although a direct causal relationship between autoimmune responses and steroid insensitivity has not been established, this study demonstrates the pathogenicity of the sputum autoantibodies, leading to heightened eosinophil activity, which is a steroid-unresponsive event. This is further corroborated by observations by Kita and coworkers[59] of nonspecific IgG, as well as ragweed-specific IgG (isolated from the sera of atopic subjects),[60] inducing eosinophil degranulation that could not be inhibited ex vivo by physiologically relevant doses of dexamethasone. In addition, the steroid-sparing clinical benefits of classic autoimmune drugs, such as azathioprine, methotrexate, and so forth, were documented in a group of 11 prednisone-dependent eosinophilic asthmatics with histologic evidence of lung granulomas.[61] These granulomas had cellular evidence of plasmacytoid cells and lymphocytes, representative of possible B-cell clusters formed as a physiologic response to unresolved chronic inflammation. Because autoantibodies were not evaluated in the study, an autoimmune type anomaly can only be speculated. Although this is an emerging concept with few available reports, local autoimmune responses in severe asthma airways could be a potential mechanism contributing to steroid insensitivity and persistence of eosinophilic luminal activity.

Recurrent infections

One of the phenotypes of asthma is characterized by mixed granulocytic sputum; that is, a raised total cell count (>10–15 million cells/g of sputum) and increased neutrophil percentage (>65%), indicating infection and, concurrently, increased eosinophil percentage (>3%) unsuppressed by current maintenance GCSs (high-dose, inhaled, and/or oral) and poor lung function.[62] The neutrophilia usually represents airway infections and the eosinophilia represents steroid insensitivity. As recently reviewed,[56] airway infections (usually bacterial) may upregulate micro-RNA 9 or 21, inhibit protein phosphatase A2, and consequently increase the activity of kinases, such as phosphoinositide 3-kinase (PI3K) and c-Jun N-terminal kinase (JNK), which may phosphorylate the glucocorticosteroid receptor. This can lead to inefficient nuclear translocation and observed steroid insensitivity.[63,64] Evidently, high endotoxin content in sputum is associated with impaired lung function response to oral GCS therapy.[65] Finally, peripheral blood mononuclear cells isolated from severe eosinophilic asthmatics with recurrent infections showed increased PI3K activity, decreased nuclear histone deacetylase (HDAC), and decreased expression of scavenger receptors on monocyte-derived macrophages, indicating susceptibility to infections.[66] It is thus currently difficult to ascertain whether recurrent infections lead to the observed GCS insensitivity via micro-RNA dysregulation or whether disease-driven changes in PI3K activity and HDAC lead to simultaneous GCS insensitivity and susceptibility to infections (see **Fig. 2**).

CLINICAL INSIGHTS: PERSISTENT AIRWAY EOSINOPHILIA AND RESPONSE TO NOVEL THERAPIES

The understanding of the underlying immunobiology of eosinophilic pathways has driven innovation and emergence of targeted treatment strategies. However, within the phenotype of eosinophilic asthma, there exists heterogeneity that is most evident from recent transcriptomic studies,[67] the diverse clinical responses to maintenance therapy, and the novel biologics currently marketed (or in clinical trials). Thus, endotyping or assessing the underlying pathways most relevant to the disease severity (see **Fig. 1**) has become crucial to classifying patients and determining the most appropriate choice of adjunct therapy.[68] mAb therapies targeting signaling molecules, such as IL-5 and IL-13, or IL-5Rα and IL-4Rα, are projected to mostly benefit those asthmatics who remain symptomatic (with airway eosinophilia) despite being on maximal GCS treatment.

Targeting T Helper Cell Type 2 Cytokines: Effect on In Situ Eosinophilopoiesis

Discordance between the systemic versus luminal antieosinophil effect of anti–IL-5 therapy indicates alternative mechanisms of in situ eosinophilic inflammation that, when unsuppressed, contribute to the ongoing clinical symptoms.[26] Administration of 750 mg intravenous (IV) mepolizumab to subjects with eosinophil-driven asthma (evidence of sputum eosinophils despite oral corticosteroid therapy) significantly reduced both blood and sputum eosinophils and allowed significant reduction in maintenance prednisone, improved asthma control and reduction in exacerbations.[69,70] In comparison, the clinical effect was modest with a 100 mg subcutaneous (SC) dose, though a consistent depletion of blood eosinophils has been documented in all phase IIIb studies (data on airway eosinophils is not available).[71–73] The reduction in exacerbation was only approximately 50% in the moderate-to-severe population[71] and 32% in the very severe eosinophilic group.[73] The effect of the low-dose therapy on airway eosinophils is available from a small Canadian substudy in which subjects who remained uncontrolled on 100 mg SC mepolizumab showed increased sputum eosinophils (>3%), albeit a significant decline in blood eosinophils.[31] This was not surprising because the seminal study reported in 2003 by Flood-Page et al.[60] showed that high-dose mepolizumab (3 monthly infusions of 750 mg IV) allowed only partial amelioration of airway eosinophils. Up to 55% decrease in airway eosinophils, 52% decrease in bone marrow eosinophils, and total depletion of blood eosinophils were reported. The study also confirmed minimal effect on airway eosinophil activity (assessed by reduction in immunostaining of major basic protein on the bronchial mucosal tissue).[60]

With respect to progenitor biology, in the initial investigations, mepolizumab arrested the maturation of eosinophils in bone marrow, depleted circulating eosinophils, and reduced the number of EoPs in the bronchial mucosa.[73] Indeed, the significant reduction in mature blood eosinophils consistently observed with both low doses and high doses of mepolizumab could be attributed to the maturation arrest of eosinophil lineage at the myelocyte and metamyelocyte stages. However, no effect was documented on early eosinophilic progenitors (CD34$^+$/IL-5Rα mRNA$^+$, or Eo/B-CFU) within the bone marrow. Nonetheless, there was partial reduction in CD34$^+$/IL-5Rα mRNA$^+$ in the bronchial mucosa.[73] In contrast, a recent study documented a significant increase in Eo/B-CFUs from cells derived from subjects who were treated with 100 mg SC mepolizumab but no change in the numbers of sputum EoPs posttreatment.[31] Finally, the same study showed subjects uncontrolled on 100 mg SC mepolizumab showed increased numbers of ILC2s in the sputum with increased intracellular staining for IL-5 and IL-13.[49] These observations suggest that patients who do not respond to lower dose of mepolizumab are likely to have, in addition to systemically derived IL-5, local derived source of IL-5 which are not effectively neutralized and could further promote in situ eosinophilopoiesis. In those subjects who remained suboptimally controlled and who continued to have persistent sputum eosinophilia, a higher dose of an anti–IL-5 mAb (in the form of weight-adjusted (3 mg/kg), IV, reslizumab) was administered that reduced sputum eosinophils and sputum EPX (a marker of eosinophil activity).[74] Furthermore, reduction in airway eosinophilopoietic factors, such as IL-5 and EoPs, were associated with improvement in asthma control and were better predictors of clinical response to IL-5 therapy than blood eosinophils.[74] This further suggested that IL-5–driven in situ eosinophilopoiesis is important for persistence of airway eosinophilia and, therefore, sputum-derived biomarkers are critical for selecting and monitoring appropriate biologic therapy.[74]

Finally, with respect to targeting the IL-4 and IL-13 pathway, dupilumab (anti–IL-4Rα mAb) was shown to reduce rate of asthma exacerbations, improve lung function, and decrease levels of type 2 inflammation (Fe$_{NO}$, TARC, eotaxin-3, and IgE) in subjects with moderate to severe eosinophilic asthma.[75] Though IL-4 and IL-13 play key roles in priming migration of eosinophils and EoPs to airways (see **Fig. 1**), currently there are no in vivo data on severe asthma and investigations are underway.

Targeting T Helper Cell Type 2 Cytokines: Effect on In Situ Autoinflammatory Processes

One of the treatment effects observed by Mukherjee and colleagues[74] was significant reduction in autoantibodies in subjects post-treatment with reslizumab, unlike that after mepolizumab. An associated increase in anti-EPX IgG and ANAs, with reduction in forced expiratory volume in 1 second (FEV_1) and worsening asthma, was observed in a prednisone-dependent eosinophilic asthmatic during an ongoing 100 mg SC mepolizumab treatment. Molecular studies revealed increased sputum IL-5, blood IL-5[+] ILC2 cells, along with high titers of anti-EPX IgG, ANAs, and BAFF. Treatment with IV immunoglobulin as an autoantibody mopping-up strategy improved lung function and decreased the autoantibody titers.[76] Presence of immunoglobulin-bound IL-5 in the sputum of subjects receiving low-dose mepolizumab with a simultaneous increase in free IL-5 and IgG autoantibodies[74,76] was suggestive of possible immune complex aggregation and subsequent inflammation. These immune complexes formed between the cytokine and the mAb, in an event in which inadequate levels of drug reach the target tissues, can increase the in vivo potency of the bound cytokine. Moreover, in a complexed form, the active sites of cytokines are prevented from in vivo degradation and hence increase the bioavailability in target tissues.[77] This is not a new concept but instead a phenomenon that has been demonstrated earlier in several in vivo studies (**Table 1**). For example, in hepatitis C virus–induced vasculitis, low-dose IL-2 therapy with consequent IL-2 or anti–IL-2 immune complexes activated ILC2 to stimulate IL-5 production, leading to a rare eosinophilia.[78] Interestingly, there was simultaneous increase in IL-5[+], ILC2s, sputum IL-5, and immunoglobulin-bound IL-5 in a subject who experienced worsening asthma with low-dose anti–IL-5 therapy.[76] The role of complement proteins and the exact mechanism of action require detailed investigation.

Currently, benralizumab, an anti–IL-5Rα afucosylated mAb, which results in a natural killer cell-mediated antibody-directed cytotoxicity,[79] is a logical therapeutic approach to target cells capable of producing IL-5 and supporting the in situ mechanisms (see **Fig. 1**). This strategy has proven to result in a greater reduction in oral glucocorticosteroids and a 55% reduction in asthma exacerbations in subjects with severe steroid-dependent asthma with an elevated blood eosinophil count ($\geq$150 cells/mm^3),[80] as well as decreasing mature eosinophils, EoPs, IL-5Rα[+], and ILC2s (but not total ILC2s), both systemically and locally,[81] within the airways. Because the drug targets the receptor, the possibility of immune complex formation and associated inflammatory complications is low. However, reduction in local autoantibodies (anti-EPX IgG) was not consistent in all subjects who received the drug.

Targeting Alarmins and Other Inflammatory Mediators

In addition to Th2 cytokines, there are other molecular targets relevant to the asthma biology that are being clinically investigated for therapeutic intervention, such as the Th2 alarmins (eg, TSLP) and the CRTH2 receptor. Although tezepelumab,[82] a mAb against TSLP,[83] and fevipiprant, a prostaglandin D2 receptor agonist,[84] were shown to reduce sputum eosinophils and improve symptoms in subjects, there is no evidence of the mechanism of action of ameliorating the local eosinophilopoietic processes.

Table 1
Outcomes in studies with cytokine: anticytokine monoclonal antibody complex

Cytokine and Known Effector Function	Animal Studies			Relevance to the Current Concept Under Review
	Animal Model	Administration (Dosage)	Observation	
IL-2 Growth factor for T cells, proliferation, and differentiation[85]	BALB/c (murine allergic inflammation model)	IL-2:anti-IL-2 antibody complex (1:10), IP	Expansion of T regs in the airways following extraneous challenge and suppression of inflammation, otherwise not observed with recombinant IL-2 or the anti-IL-2 antibody alone	Increased biological activity of IL-2 on administration of the IC
IL-2 Lin⁻ CD25⁺ innate lymphoid cells (ILC2s) proliferate in presence of IL-2[86]	Red5 mice (IL-5 reporter mice) backcrossed to C57BL/6	IL-2: anti–IL-2 mAb complex, IP	5-fold increase in ILC2s, which were IL-5⁺ and subsequent increase in eosinophils	Increased in vivo potency with increased downstream effector mechanisms
IL-4 IgE and IgG₁ production by B cells[87]	BALB/c	Coadministration of exogenous IL-4 and anti–IL-4 IgG₁, IP	3-fold increase in IgE production in mice treated with 2.5 μg IL-4⁺ 40 μg anti–IL-4 mAb in comparison with mice treated with IL-4 alone This was reversed at the highest concentration of 100 μg/mL mAb	Increased in vivo biological activity of IL-4 on IgE and IgG₁ production with coadministration of optimal anti–IL-4 mAb
IL-4 IL-3[77] Mucosal mast cell response	BALB/c	5 μg IL-4⁺ 30 μg anti–IL-4 mAb 20 μg IL-3⁺ 100 μg anti–IL-3 mAb Or combination of ICs, IV	Immune complex formed by IL-4 and neutralizing anti–IL-4 mAb increased mucosal mast cells by 16-fold compared with the individual cytokines Combination of ICs induced an additive effect	Increased in vivo potency of cytokines when aggregated in immune complexes due to increased in vivo half-life
IL-7 B-cell development and increase[77]	BALB/c	5μg IL-7⁺ 25 μg anti–IL-7 mAb, IV	Increase in B-cell production in bone marrow and consequent increase of B220⁺ IgM⁻ IgD⁻ B cells in spleen	IC of IL-7:anti:IL-7 allowed longer time in circulation and directly increased its biological activity
IL-7 Survival and proliferation of T cells[88]	C57BL/6	1.5 μg IL-7⁺ 7.5 μg anti–IL-7 mAb	Increased stimulation of T cells in the secondary lymphoid organs Increased proliferation of T cells	Increased in vivo life span of IL-7 IL-7:anti–IL-7 engaged the neonatal FcRn and reduced clearance Increased cytokine availability to IL-7R

Human Studies

Therapy	Target Cytokine	Disease	Relevance to Current Concept Under Review	Clinical Relevance
IL-2[89]	Phase 1 or 2 0.33 MIU/d, 1 MIU/d, or 3 MIU/d for a 5-d course dosage of IL-2	Type 1 diabetes	Dose-dependent increase in IL-5 and eosinophils in some subjects Nonserious adverse events in treatment group	Increase in Tregs (primary outcome) Eosinophilia was an unexplained side effect and investigated later by Van Gool et al[86]
Mepolizumab[90]	Anti–IL-5 IgG$_{1\kappa}$ 750 mg IV	Eosinophilic esophagitis (severe n = 4)	Increased plasma level of IL-5 and eotaxin-3 after dosing Though clinical improvement was logged, increase in the target cytokine raised concern	All 4 subjects showed significant clinical improvement
Mepolizumab[91]	Anti–IL-5 IgG$_{1\kappa}$ 750 mg IV	Hypereosinophilic disorders (n = 18) Eosinophilic esophagitis (n = 6)	Increased IL-5 bound to Ig fractions immunoprecipitated from blood Increased T-cell stimulations and IL-5α^+ cells in treated vs placebo	Modest improvement in subjects Did not correlate with IL-5 levels

This is not an exhaustive list.
Abbreviations: IC, immune complex; IP, intraperitoneal; IV, intravenous.

SUMMARY

Airway eosinophils contribute significantly to luminal obstruction and symptoms in asthma. As asthma becomes more severe, in addition to the classic type 2 inflammatory cascade–mediated process of eosinophil recruitment into the lung, additional processes, such as in situ eosinophilopoiesis and lung-compartmentalized autoimmune responses, may contribute to the persistence of airway eosinophilia. Glucocorticosteroid insensitivity, exaggerated by several mechanisms, including autoimmune responses, may further contribute to airway eosinophilia. These processes are relevant when choosing the appropriate biologic to control eosinophilia in patients with severe asthma.

REFERENCES

1. Kay AB. The early history of the eosinophil. Clin Exp Allergy 2015;45(3):575–82.
2. Brown HM. Treatment of chronic asthma with prednisolone; significance of eosinophils in the sputum. Lancet 1958;13(2):1245–7.
3. Hargreave FE, Nair P. The definition and diagnosis of asthma. Clin Exp Allergy 2009;39(11):1652–8.
4. D'Silva L, Hassan N, Wang HY, et al. Heterogeneity of bronchitis in airway diseases in tertiary care clinical practice. Can Respir J 2011;18(3):144–8.
5. Nair P, Dasgupta A, Brightling CE, et al. How to diagnose and phenotype asthma. Clin Chest Med 2012;33(3):445–57.
6. Papi A, Brightling C, Pedersen SE, et al. Asthma. Lancet 2018. https://doi.org/10.1016/S0140–6736(17)33311-1.
7. Chung KF, Wenzel SE, Brozek JL, et al. International ERS/ATS guidelines on definition, evaluation and treatment of severe asthma. Eur Respir J 2014;43(2):343–73.
8. van Veen IH, Ten Brinke A, Gauw SA, et al. Consistency of sputum eosinophilia in difficult-to-treat asthma: a 5-year follow-up study. J Allergy Clin Immunol 2009;124(3):615–7, 617.e1–2.
9. Mukherjee M, Nair P. Blood or sputum eosinophils to guide asthma therapy? Lancet Respir Med 2015;3(11):824–5.
10. Lacy P, Moqbel R. Immune effector functions of eosinophils in allergic airway inflammation. Curr Opin Allergy Clin Immunol 2001;1(1):79–84.
11. Hogan SP, Rosenberg HF, Moqbel R, et al. Eosinophils: biological properties and role in health and disease. Clin Exp Allergy 2008;38(5):709–50.
12. Shi HZ. Eosinophils function as antigen-presenting cells. J Leukoc Biol 2004;76(3):520–7.
13. Davoine F, Lacy P. Eosinophil cytokines, chemokines, and growth factors: emerging roles in immunity. Front Immunol 2014;5:570.
14. Lacy P, Moqbel R. Signalling and degranulation. In: Lee JJ, Rosenberg HF, editors. Eosinophils in health and disease, vol. 1. San Diego (CA): Academic Press (Elsevier); 2013. p. 206–18.
15. Willetts L, Ochkur SI, Jacobsen EA, et al. Eosinophil shape change and secretion. In: Walsh GM, editor. Eosinophils: methods and protocols. New York: Springer; 2014. p. 111–28.
16. Ueki S, Melo RC, Ghiran I, et al. Eosinophil extracellular DNA trap cell death mediates lytic release of free secretion-competent eosinophil granules in humans. Blood 2013;121(11):2074–83.
17. Persson C, Uller L. Theirs but to die and do: primary lysis of eosinophils and free eosinophil granules in asthma. Am J Respir Crit Care Med 2014;189(6):628–33.

18. Nair P, Ochkur SI, Protheroe C, et al. Eosinophil peroxidase in sputum represents a unique biomarker of airway eosinophilia. Allergy 2013;68(9):1177–84.

19. Maltby S, McNagny KM. Introduction: eosinophilopoiesis. In: Lee JJ, Rosenberg HF, editors. Eosinophils in health and disease. San Diego (CA): Academic Press (Elsevier); 2013. p. 73–5.

20. Salter BM, Sehmi R. Hematopoietic processes in eosinophilic asthma. Chest 2017;152(2):410–6.

21. Rothenberg ME, Hogan SP. The eosinophil. Annu Rev Immunol 2006;24(1):147–74.

22. Bochner BS, Schleimer RP. The role of adhesion molecules in human eosinophil and basophil recruitment. J Allergy Clin Immunol 1994;94(3 Pt 1):427–38 [quiz: 439].

23. Zimmermann N, Hershey GK, Foster PS, et al. Chemokines in asthma: cooperative interaction between chemokines and IL-13. J Allergy Clin Immunol 2003;111(2):227–42 [quiz: 243].

24. Rankin SM, Conroy DM, Williams TJ. Eotaxin and eosinophil recruitment: implications for human disease. Mol Med Today 2000;6(1):20–7.

25. Sanderson CJ. Interleukin-5, eosinophils, and disease. Blood 1992;79(12):3101–9.

26. Mukherjee M, Sehmi R, Nair P. Anti-IL5 therapy for asthma and beyond. World Allergy Organ J 2014;7(1):32.

27. Kim YK, Uno M, Hamilos DL, et al. Immunolocalization of CD34 in nasal polyposis. Effect of topical corticosteroids. Am J Respir Cell Mol Biol 1999;20(3):388–97.

28. Cameron L, Christodoulopoulos P, Lavigne F, et al. Evidence for local eosinophil differentiation within allergic nasal mucosa: inhibition with soluble IL-5 receptor. J Immunol 2000;164(3):1538–45.

29. Sehmi R, Howie K, Sutherland DR, et al. Increased levels of CD34+ hemopoietic progenitor cells in atopic subjects. Am J Respir Cell Mol Biol 1996;15(5):645–55.

30. Robinson DS, Damia R, Zeibecoglou K, et al. CD34(+)/interleukin-5Ralpha messenger RNA+ cells in the bronchial mucosa in asthma: potential airway eosinophil progenitors. Am J Respir Cell Mol Biol 1999;20(1):9–13.

31. Sehmi R, Smith SG, Kjarsgaard M, et al. Role of local eosinophilopoietic processes in the development of airway eosinophilia in prednisone-dependent severe asthma. Clin Exp Allergy 2016;46(6):793–802.

32. Neighbour H, Boulet LP, Lemiere C, et al. Safety and efficacy of an oral CCR3 antagonist in patients with asthma and eosinophilic bronchitis: a randomized, placebo-controlled clinical trial. Clin Exp Allergy 2014;44(4):508–16.

33. Wills-Karp M, Finkelman FD. Untangling the complex web of IL-4- and IL-13-mediated signaling pathways. Sci Signal 2008;1(51):pe55.

34. Zhu Z, Homer RJ, Wang Z, et al. Pulmonary expression of interleukin-13 causes inflammation, mucus hypersecretion, subepithelial fibrosis, physiologic abnormalities, and eotaxin production. J Clin Invest 1999;103(6):779–88.

35. Wills-Karp M. Interleukin-13 in asthma pathogenesis. Curr Allergy Asthma Rep 2004;4(2):123–31.

36. Dorman SC, Babirad I, Post J, et al. Progenitor egress from the bone marrow after allergen challenge: role of stromal cell-derived factor 1alpha and eotaxin. J Allergy Clin Immunol 2005;115(3):501–7.

37. Punia N, Smith S, Thomson JV, et al. Interleukin-4 and interleukin-13 prime migrational responses of haemopoietic progenitor cells to stromal cell-derived factor-1α. Clin Exp Allergy 2012;42(2):255–64.

38. Mitchell PD, O'Byrne PM. Biologics and the lung: TSLP and other epithelial cell-derived cytokines in asthma. Pharmacol Ther 2017;169:104–12.

39. Guy GB, Tania M, Ken RB. Eosinophils in the spotlight: eosinophilic airway inflammation in nonallergic asthma. Nat Med 2013;19(8):977–9.

40. Prefontaine D, Nadigel J, Chouiali F, et al. Increased IL-33 expression by epithelial cells in bronchial asthma. J Allergy Clin Immunol 2010;125(3):752–4.

41. Shikotra A, Choy DF, Ohri CM, et al. Increased expression of immunoreactive thymic stromal lymphopoietin in patients with severe asthma. J Allergy Clin Immunol 2012;129(1):104–11.e1-9.

42. Ying S, O'Connor B, Ratoff J, et al. Thymic stromal lymphopoietin expression is increased in asthmatic airways and correlates with expression of Th2-attracting chemokines and disease severity. J Immunol 2005;174(12):8183–90.

43. Salter BMA, Smith SG, Mukherjee M, et al. Human bronchial epithelial cell-derived factors from severe asthmatic subjects stimulate eosinophil differentiation. Am J Respir Cell Mol Biol 2017;58(1):99–106.

44. Smith SG, Gugilla A, Mukherjee M, et al. Thymic stromal lymphopoietin and IL-33 modulate migration of hematopoietic progenitor cells in patients with allergic asthma. J Allergy Clin Immunol 2015;135(6):1594–602.

45. Spits H, Di Santo JP. The expanding family of innate lymphoid cells: regulators and effectors of immunity and tissue remodeling. Nat Immunol 2011;12(1):21–7.

46. Walker JA, McKenzie AN. Development and function of group 2 innate lymphoid cells. Curr Opin Immunol 2013;25(2):148–55.

47. Kim HY, Chang YJ, Subramanian S, et al. Innate lymphoid cells responding to IL-33 mediate airway hyperreactivity independently of adaptive immunity. J Allergy Clin Immunol 2012;129(1):216–27.e1-6.

48. Barlow JL, Peel S, Fox J, et al. IL-33 is more potent than IL-25 in provoking IL-13-producing nuocytes (type 2 innate lymphoid cells) and airway contraction. J Allergy Clin Immunol 2013;132(4):933–41.

49. Smith SG, Chen R, Kjarsgaard M, et al. Increased numbers of activated group 2 innate lymphoid cells in the airways of patients with severe asthma and persistent airway eosinophilia. J Allergy Clin Immunol 2016;137(1):75–86.e8.

50. Lambrecht BN, Hammad H. The airway epithelium in asthma. Nat Med 2012; 18(5):684–92.

51. Holtzman MJ, Byers DE, Alexander-Brett J, et al. The role of airway epithelial cells and innate immune cells in chronic respiratory disease. Nat Rev Immunol 2014; 14(10):686–98.

52. Christianson CA, Goplen NP, Zafar I, et al. Persistence of asthma requires multiple feedback circuits involving type 2 innate lymphoid cells and IL-33. J Allergy Clin Immunol 2015;136(1):59–68.e4.

53. Lazaar AL, Panettieri RA Jr. Airway smooth muscle as a regulator of immune responses and bronchomotor tone. Clin Chest Med 2006;27(1):53–69, vi.

54. Panettieri RA Jr. Airway smooth muscle: an immunomodulatory cell. J Allergy Clin Immunol 2002;110(6 Suppl):S269–74.

55. Fanat AI, Thomson JV, Radford K, et al. Human airway smooth muscle promotes eosinophil differentiation. Clin Exp Allergy 2009;39(7):1009–17.

56. Mukherjee M, Svenningsen S, Nair P. Glucocorticosteroid subsensitivity and asthma severity. Curr Opin Pulm Med 2017;23(1):78–88.

57. Keenan CR, Radojicic D, Li M, et al. Heterogeneity in mechanisms influencing glucocorticoid sensitivity: the need for a systems biology approach to treatment of glucocorticoid-resistant inflammation. Pharmacol Ther 2015;150:81–93.

58. Mukherjee M, Bulir DC, Radford K, et al. Sputum autoantibodies in patients with severe eosinophilic asthma. J Allergy Clin Immunol 2018;141(4):1269–79.

59. Kita H, Abu-Ghazaleh R, Sanderson CJ, et al. Effect of steroids on immunoglobulin-induced eosinophil degranulation. J Allergy Clin Immunol 1991;87(1 Pt 1):70–7.

60. Flood-Page PT, Menzies-Gow AN, Kay AB, et al. Eosinophil's role remains uncertain as anti–interleukin-5 only partially depletes numbers in asthmatic airway. Am J Respir Crit Care Med 2003;167(2):199–204.

61. Wenzel SE, Vitari CA, Shende M, et al. Asthmatic granulomatosis: a novel disease with asthmatic and granulomatous features. Am J Respir Crit Care Med 2012; 186(6):501–7.

62. Chu DK, Al-Garawi A, Llop-Guevara A, et al. Therapeutic potential of anti-IL-6 therapies for granulocytic airway inflammation in asthma. Allergy Asthma Clin Immunol 2015;11(1):1–6.

63. Li JJ, Tay HL, Maltby S, et al. MicroRNA-9 regulates steroid-resistant airway hyperresponsiveness by reducing protein phosphatase 2A activity. J Allergy Clin Immunol 2015;136(2):462–73.

64. Kim RY, Horvat JC, Pinkerton JW, et al. MicroRNA-21 drives severe, steroid-insensitive experimental asthma by amplifying phosphoinositide 3-kinase-mediated suppression of histone deacetylase 2. J Allergy Clin Immunol 2017;139(2): 519–32.

65. McSharry C, Spears M, Chaudhuri R, et al. Increased sputum endotoxin levels are associated with an impaired lung function response to oral steroids in asthmatic patients. J Allergy Clin Immunol 2014;134(5):1068–75.

66. Zuccaro L, Cox A, Pray C, et al. Histone deacetylase activity and recurrent bacterial bronchitis in severe eosinophilic asthma. Allergy 2016;71(4):571–5.

67. Hekking P-P, Loza MJ, Pavlidis S, et al. Pathway discovery using transcriptomic profiles in adult-onset severe asthma. J Allergy Clin Immunol 2018;141(4): 1280–90.

68. Svenningsen S, Nair P. Asthma endotypes and an overview of targeted therapy for asthma. Front Med (Lausanne) 2017;4(158):158.

69. Haldar P, Brightling CE, Hargadon B, et al. Mepolizumab and exacerbations of refractory eosinophilic asthma. N Engl J Med 2009;360(10):973–84.

70. Nair P, Pizzichini MM, Kjarsgaard M, et al. Mepolizumab for prednisone-dependent asthma with sputum eosinophilia. N Engl J Med 2009;360(10): 985–93.

71. Ortega HG, Liu MC, Pavord ID, et al. Mepolizumab treatment in patients with severe eosinophilic asthma. N Engl J Med 2014;371(13):1198–207.

72. Bel EH, Wenzel SE, Thompson PJ, et al. Oral glucocorticoid-sparing effect of mepolizumab in eosinophilic asthma. N Engl J Med 2014;371(13):1189–97.

73. Menzies-Gow A, Flood-Page P, Sehmi R, et al. Anti-IL-5 (mepolizumab) therapy induces bone marrow eosinophil maturational arrest and decreases eosinophil progenitors in the bronchial mucosa of atopic asthmatics. J Allergy Clin Immunol 2003;111(4):714–9.

74. Mukherjee M, Aleman Paramo F, Kjarsgaard M, et al. Weight-adjusted intravenous reslizumab in severe asthma with inadequate response to fixed-dose subcutaneous mepolizumab. Am J Respir Crit Care Med 2018;197(1):38–46.

75. Wenzel S, Ford L, Pearlman D, et al. Dupilumab in persistent asthma with elevated eosinophil levels. N Engl J Med 2013;368(26):2455–66.

76. Mukherjee M, Lim HF, Thomas S, et al. Airway autoimmune responses in severe eosinophilic asthma following low-dose Mepolizumab therapy. Allergy Asthma Clin Immunol 2017;13:2.

77. Finkelman FD, Madden KB, Morris SC, et al. Anti-cytokine antibodies as carrier proteins. Prolongation of in vivo effects of exogenous cytokines by injection of cytokine-anti-cytokine antibody complexes. J Immunol 1993;151(3):1235–44.

78. Saadoun D, Rosenzwajg M, Joly F, et al. Regulatory T-cell responses to low-dose interleukin-2 in HCV-induced vasculitis. N Engl J Med 2011;365(22):2067–77.

79. Kolbeck R, Kozhich A, Koike M, et al. MEDI-563, a humanized anti-IL-5 receptor alpha mAb with enhanced antibody-dependent cell-mediated cytotoxicity function. J Allergy Clin Immunol 2010;125(6):1344–53.e2.

80. Nair P, Wenzel S, Rabe KF, et al. Oral glucocorticoid-sparing effect of benralizumab in severe asthma. N Engl J Med 2017;376(25):2448–58.

81. Sehmi R, Lim HF, Mukherjee M, et al. Benralizumab attenuates airway eosinophilia in prednisone-dependent asthma. J Allergy Clin Immunol 2018;141(4):1529–32.e8.

82. Corren J, Parnes JR, Wang L, et al. Tezepelumab in adults with uncontrolled asthma. N Engl J Med 2017;377(10):936–46.

83. Gauvreau GM, O'Byrne PM, Boulet LP, et al. Effects of an anti-TSLP antibody on allergen-induced asthmatic responses. N Engl J Med 2014;370(22):2102–10.

84. Gonem S, Berair R, Singapuri A, et al. Fevipiprant, a prostaglandin D2 receptor 2 antagonist, in patients with persistent eosinophilic asthma: a single-centre, randomised, double-blind, parallel-group, placebo-controlled trial. Lancet Respir Med 2016;4(9):699–707.

85. Wilson MS, Pesce JT, Ramalingam TR, et al. Suppression of murine allergic airway disease by IL-2:anti-IL-2 monoclonal antibody-induced regulatory T cells. J Immunol 2008;181(10):6942–54.

86. Van Gool F, Molofsky AB, Morar MM, et al. Interleukin-5–producing group 2 innate lymphoid cells control eosinophilia induced by interleukin-2 therapy. Blood 2014;124(24):3572–6.

87. Sato TA, Widmer MB, Finkelman FD, et al. Recombinant soluble murine IL-4 receptor can inhibit or enhance IgE responses in vivo. J Immunol 1993;150(7):2717–23.

88. Martin CE, van Leeuwen EMM, Im SJ, et al. IL-7/anti–IL-7 mAb complexes augment cytokine potency in mice through association with IgG-Fc and by competition with IL-7R. Blood 2013;121(22):4484–92.

89. Hartemann A, Bensimon G, Payan CA, et al. Low-dose interleukin 2 in patients with type 1 diabetes: a phase 1/2 randomised, double-blind, placebo-controlled trial. Lancet Diabetes Endocrinol 2013;1(4):295–305.

90. Stein ML, Collins MH, Villanueva JM, et al. Anti–IL-5 (mepolizumab) therapy for eosinophilic esophagitis. J Allergy Clin Immunol 2006;118(6):1312–9.

91. Stein ML, Villanueva JM, Buckmeier BK, et al. Anti–IL-5 (mepolizumab) therapy reduces eosinophil activation ex vivo and increases IL-5 and IL-5 receptor levels. J Allergy Clin Immunol 2008;121(6):1473–83.e4.

Molecular Endotypes Contribute to the Heterogeneity of Asthma

Erwin W. Gelfand, MD, Michaela Schedel, PhD*

KEYWORDS

- Asthma • Endotypes • Biomarker • Transcriptomics • Sputum • Epithelium
- Human rhinovirus infection • Steroid-resistant asthma

KEY POINTS

- Molecular endotyping in sputum, airway epithelial cells, and blood increases our understanding of the clinical heterogeneity of asthma.
- Varying genes and pathways contribute to the development and progression of asthma depending on the tissue, trigger, and disease status.
- Endotyping can be a screening tool to identify useful biomarkers of disease, risk assessment, and treatment response.
- Well-characterized, longitudinal cohorts are necessary to define critical endotypes to advance the diagnosis, classification, and treatment of asthmatic patients.

Asthma is one of the most common chronic diseases. Commonly, clinical measurements have been used to diagnose and manage the disease. Depending on symptom severity, guideline-supported approaches recommend inhaled corticosteroids (ICS) for disease control and β2-agonists for disease rescue. However, this one-size-fits-all approach to disease management has been called into question, particularly in light of the increasing recognition that asthma is heterogeneous, one that is not stable over time but responsive to ever-changing environmental stimuli, and corticosteroids (CS) may not always be effective. Defining subgroups of asthmatic patients based on clinical parameters and cluster analyses incorporating lung function, medication usage, and other clinical variables has been challenging. Identification of biomarkers that associate with these subgroups have centered around measurements of airway inflammation,[1] levels of exhaled nitric oxide (FeNO),[2] and serum periostin levels.[3,4] Although useful, these nonmolecular biomarkers provide limited resolution of disease

Conflict of Interest Statement: The authors have no conflicts of interest to declare.

Division of Cell Biology, Department of Pediatrics, National Jewish Health, 1400 Jackson Street, Denver, CO 80206, USA

* Corresponding author.

E-mail address: schedelm@njhealth.org

Immunol Allergy Clin N Am 38 (2018) 655–665

https://doi.org/10.1016/j.iac.2018.06.008

0889-8561/18/© 2018 Elsevier Inc. All rights reserved.

immunology.theclinics.com

subgroups and little information regarding the underlying pathobiology of the disease in individual subjects. In contrast, molecular data generated from asthmatic patients hold great promise in the delineation of pathobiological subgroups, bioactive pathways, and true disease endotypes. In particular, the ability to query the entire transcriptome in a single assay (microarray technology and/or RNA-sequencing [RNA-seq]) has provided a powerful tool to comprehensively define the molecular dysfunction of a tissue at a patient level and then relate these molecular patterns to clinical traits. The complex cause of asthma defined by endotyping of a single tissue will only provide a partial picture of the disease. Reflecting this, expression studies of sputum, airway, and blood have all contributed significant information to our understanding of asthma pathobiology; but results have been discordant. Additionally, the dynamic nature of the transcriptome requires studies examining tissues at different developmental and disease stages, environmental exposures or infection status which will contribute unique information about asthma. Collectively, these studies have and will continue to provide a more comprehensive picture of asthma endotypes, associated biomarkers, and potential pharmacologic targets, as discussed later.

MOLECULAR ENDOTYPES CORRELATE WITH ASTHMA PHENOTYPES USING SPUTUM TRANSCRIPTOMICS

Most asthmatic patients have some degree of chronic inflammation of the airways. Analyses of induced sputum cells offer a noninvasive technique to collect and quantify inflammatory cell populations in the airways of asthmatic patients. To a large extent the composition of these samples includes both innate (macrophages, neutrophils, eosinophils, innate lymphocytes) and adaptive immune cells (CD4+ and CD8+ lymphocytes). Although sputum eosinophilic airway inflammation in asthmatic patients is the most prevalent, asthmatic patients can be classified into 4 subgroups based on the cell composition at a particular point in time: eosinophilic, neutrophilic, mixed granulocytic (eosinophilic and neutrophilic), and pauci-granulocytic (normal or near normal eosinophil/neutrophil numbers).[5,6] Compared with the pauci-granulocytic phenotype, eosinophilic, neutrophilic, and mixed granulocytic asthmatic patients exhibit poorer lung function.[5] Severe asthma has tended to associate with increased neutrophil numbers rather than eosinophils in their airways (neutrophilic asthma), a phenomenon typically related to nonallergic asthma and thought to be triggered by particulates in the air, pollution, viruses, or bacteria.[7] Important in understanding this inflammatory cell heterogeneity is the impact of drugs. Whereas eosinophils seem to be CS-sensitive and readily undergoing apoptosis, neutrophils seem to be insensitive to CS.[8] Although attempts have been made to track these airway inflammatory subgroups by monitoring blood granulocyte levels, this has only been partially helpful for eosinophilic disease and poorly for neutrophilic asthma.

Studies have been extended to the molecular level through generation of gene expression profiles from sputum cells and peripheral blood to determine whether the clinical heterogeneity of asthma is also reflected in underlying molecular pathways. Sputum microarray transcriptomic data from 100 asthmatic subjects were recently used to identify transcriptomic endotypes of asthma (TEA) clusters.[9] The expression of genes within predefined pathways was used in unsupervised clustering analyses of TEA groups based on the pathway distance between samples and resulted in 3 distinct clusters. To determine the phenotypic correlates of these TEA subgroups, clinical variables were compared: TEA cluster 1 was associated with lower prebronchodilator forced expiratory volume in the first second of inspiration (FEV1), a higher bronchodilator response, higher FeNO levels, and ICS usage; TEA cluster 2 contained individuals with prior hospitalization for asthma and no atopy history: TEA cluster 3 was enriched for patients with mild asthma, associated with better lung function, decreased FeNO, and lower ICS requirements. A similar approach was taken in asthmatic patients where both sputum and peripheral blood expression data were available. An expression signature encompassing 53 genes in the blood separated the population into clusters that closely resembled the TEA subgroups observed in the sputum. The identification and clinical characteristics of TEA clusters represented by this gene signature were largely replicated in the Asthma BioRepository for Integrative Genomic Exploration (Asthma BRIDGE) cohort. Importantly, the investigators did not find these TEA clusters to be associated with sputum inflammatory cell numbers per se, supporting the importance of molecular sputum analyses for clinical associations. Moreover, these studies suggested that blood gene expression patterns can be informative in clinically defined clustering of asthmatic patients.

Comprehensive approaches have been taken by the Unbiased Biomarkers in Prediction of Respiratory Disease Outcomes (U-BIOPRED) consortia to test if molecular differences in the sputum and other tissues, for example, blood, exist between clinically assigned groups but also to discover distinct asthma phenotypes based on endo-typic signatures. This European cohort included nonsmoking patients with severe asthma (SA), smoking/ex-smoking patients with SA, nonsmoking patients with mild/moderate asthma (MMA), and healthy nonsmoking controls.[10] One focus of this cohort study was to perform molecular phenotyping of sputum cells to define endotypes in patients with severe asthma that relate to sputum granulocytic inflammation.[11] Inflammatory cell counts revealed the highest sputum eosinophils in smoking and nonsmoking SA, whereas neutrophilic inflammation did not vary between groups. When transcriptomic profiles were compared between the 4 different subgroups, 801 transcripts were differentially expressed in nonsmoking SA versus healthy controls and 172 genes comparing nonsmoking SA with MMA, respectively. Key genes that were upregulated in the sputum of nonsmoking SA included members of the interleukin 1 (IL-1) receptor (*IL-1R*) family and the inflammasome pathway (eg, *IL1RL1, IL18R1, NLRP3, ILRL1, IL1RL2, IRAK3, IL18RAP*). When *IL-1R* and inflammasome-related genes were correlated with specific sputum granulocyte subtypes, a predominance of eosinophilic inflammation, enhanced T helper 2 (Th2) cytokine protein expression, and *IL1RL1* messenger RNA (mRNA) levels was detected. In contrast, elevated expression of *IL-1* and *IL-18R* family members, *NLRP1, NLRP3, NLRC4*, and other members of the inflammasome were associated with neutrophilic asthma. Of note, these changes were validated in the Airways Disease Endotyping for Personalized Therapeutics (ADEPT) cohort[12] but seemed specific for sputum, as similar effects were not seen in bronchial brushings or biopsies from SA in the U-BIOPRED cohort.[11] Further validation of the relevance of the NLRP3 inflammasome was provided in a model of experimental asthma. In vivo administration of the inflammasome inhibitor CRID3 prevented the development of lung allergic responses and reduced the expression of IL-1β, Th2 cytokines, and neutrophil- and eosinophil-associated chemokines. Such studies underscore the need to incorporate both human and animal studies to validate biologically relevant mechanisms and translate the clinical heterogeneity of human asthma through mechanistic understanding of the pathobiology.

Additional molecular endotying studies of sputum have focused on defining the presence or absence of type 2 cytokine-mediated airway inflammation. For example, Peters and colleagues[13] found gene expression changes of the type 2 cytokines *IL-4, IL-5*, and *IL-13* in sputum cell pellets. Moreover, they developed an algorithm to classify asthmatic patients as having type 2-high or type 2-low disease. Subjects with type 2-high disease had more severe disease and increased sputum and blood eosinophil numbers. A transcriptome-wide study was conducted to define molecular mechanisms of type 2-high and type 2-low asthma in the sputum of patients with severe disease (U-BIOPRED[10]) and identified involvement of 10 relevant pathways. These pathways included immune activation and cytokine production, regulation of cysteine-type endopeptidase activity, pattern recognition receptor signaling, response to interferon-γ, ice protease-activating factor inflammasome complex, and Nucleotide-binding, oligomerization domain like receptor signaling.[14] Moreover, this study identified interferon-, tumor necrosis factor-α-, and inflammasome-associated signatures that were associated with type 2-low, neutrophilic asthma. Pauci-granulocytic patients exhibited a molecular profile characteristic of increased mitochondrial energy metabolic pathways, with the highest expression scores for mitochondrial oxidative stress (oxidative phosphorylation) and aging.

Taken together, these studies confirm the value of molecular analyses of sputum cells to increase our understanding of the clinical heterogeneity of asthma, to delineate the varying airway inflammatory pathways in asthma, and to define useful biomarkers that associate with disease. One limitation of these studies is that they are single-point-in-time analyses and do not reflect the dynamic nature of asthma.

TRANSCRIPTOMIC PROFILES IN EPITHELIAL CELLS OF ASTHMATIC PATIENTS ARE DISTINCT FROM HEALTHY INDIVIDUALS

One potential mechanism contributing to asthma pathobiology is through disrupted epithelial barrier function of airway epithelial cells due to transcriptional reprogramming.[15,16] However, dysregulated genes and pathways involved in this signaling process are poorly understood. One of the first mechanistic studies to characterize molecular endotypes in airway epithelial brushings from asthmatic patients identified a gene signature consisting of PERIOSTIN, CLCA1, and SERPINB2 as potential markers of the IL-13–driven, CS-responsive asthma phenotype.[17] Based on the initial data, asthmatic patients with a Th2-high or a Th2-low profile were defined.[18] Key features within the Th2-high group were increased IL-5 and IL-13 levels, bronchial hyper-responsiveness, elevated serum immunoglobulin E levels, and blood and airway eosinophilia. The Th2-high group was more likely to be atopic and responsive to ICS, although this has been less consistent in other studies.[19]

A similar pattern distinguishing Th2-high versus Th2-low asthmatic patients was demonstrated in nasal epithelial cell brushings.[20] Overall, expression patterns in nasal brushings largely recapitulated changes in the airways (bronchial brushings) with an overlap of more than 90%. Hierarchic clustering analyses of nasal epithelial cells separated the Th2-high versus Th2-low group by global expression changes in 70 genes, including PERIOSTIN, CLCA1, SERPINB, IL-13, and IL-5. An IL-13–induced/Th2-high signature was also found in the sputum of asthmatic patients, although with a lower magnitude,[11] suggesting that Th2 signatures in the sputum and epithelial cells may be driven by different pathways. Identification of patients as Th2-high may predict those who would benefit from treatment specifically targeting type 2 pathways, for example, dupilumab, yet these asthmatic patients were shown to be well controlled with standard ICS treatment.

Studies analyzing paired bronchial biopsies and epithelial brushings from the same patient have shown the relationship between gene expression clusters and unique clinical signatures in patients with moderate to severe asthma (U-BIOPRED).[19] Surprisingly, none of the gene sets was significantly different in epithelial brushings from SA compared with patients with moderate asthma. In contrast, unsupervised and hierarchical clustering of bronchial biopsy transcriptomes identified 2 clusters (cluster A and cluster non-A). Cluster A was characterized by high submucosal eosinophilia and higher FeNO and oral CS use with 26 out of 42 gene sets differentially expressed. These gene sets were associated with asthma, immune, and/or inflammatory pathways. In addition, an overlapping 9-gene set signature between bronchial biopsies and epithelial brushings distinguished patients exhibiting high Th2 activation (groups 1 and 3) versus a group of non–Th2-mediated asthma subtypes (groups 2 and 4). In this study, one interesting finding was the identification of a subgroup of patients (group 1) with a unique molecular endotype associated with a Th2 signature, increased CD3[+] and CD8[+] T cells, and a CS insensitivity, which is in contrast to previous findings.[18] This group of SA who appear refractory (insensitive) to CS are a clinical challenge. One possible mechanism, as suggested here and in the authors' previous work, is through the involvement of increased numbers of CD8[+] T cells that are insensitive to CS[21,22] and can undergo transcriptional reprogramming and conversion to IL-13 production (Tc2) in an IL-4–dependent manner through an orchestrated cascade of molecular and cellular events.[23,24]

Transcriptional changes across multiple airway tissues has been investigated by combining data from epithelial brushings and airway T cells from the sputum and bronchoalveolar lavage (BAL) fluid from the same patient.[25] In sorted CD3[+] T cells, a distinct transcriptomic signature was observed when compared to epithelial brushings, while no differences were seen between T cells isolated from the BAL and sputum. The changes primarily reflected cell type differences rather than disease-related effects. As previously shown for the epithelium,[17,20,26] IL-13-response genes including PERIOSTIN, CLCA1, and SERPINB2 were differentially expressed in patients with mild asthma compared with controls.[25] In addition, mast cell mediators (CPA3, TPSAB1), inducible nitric oxide synthase, and cystatin (CST1, CST2, CST4) genes were upregulated in asthmatic patients. After CS treatment of patients with moderate asthma, mRNA levels were downregulated with the exception of cystatin genes, indicating asthma control in these patients. Interestingly, in BAL T cells, none of the genes were altered in patients with mild asthma versus controls; SCGB1A1 was the only gene with changes in patients with moderate asthma, suggesting that sputum may be more reflective of ongoing inflammation. The largest number of gene expression changes was observed in the sputum of SA, a predominantly neutrophilic phenotype, compared with controls. As predicted, some gene signatures were associated with IL-17–inducible chemokines (CXCL1, CXCL2, CXCL3, IL-8, CSF3) and neutrophil chemoattractants (IL-8, CCL3, LGALS3), whereas others were related to T cells and monocytes. The investigators concluded that an IL-13 signature was detected primarily in patients with mild asthma, whereas patients with more severe asthma were prone to neutrophilic inflammation with steroid-insensitive IL-17 transcriptomic patterns.

As suggested earlier, a major challenge is comparing molecular patterns across different studies and linking them to disease severity or phenotype. In a study mining public microarray data sets from 8 independent studies of asthmatic bronchial epithelial cells, consistent expression differences involving 159 genes in at least 5 studies that were tightly linked to lung and epithelial biology were shown.[26] Subsequent network analyses classified hubs of 12 genes involved in more than one functional pathway supporting biological relevance. In this study, PERIOSTIN was among the 12 marker genes. Surprisingly, an underlying suppression of epithelial differentiation, including insulin and Notch signaling pathways (EFNB2, FGFR1, FGFR2, INSR, IRS2, NOTCH2, TLE1, and NTRK2), was most prominent. Epithelial dedifferentiation programs were shared across the cohorts of mild, moderate, and severe asthmatic patients, which were more pronounced with increasing disease severity. Further functional validation of these findings was provided after performing RNA-seq on cultured human bronchial epithelial cells. In healthy controls versus asthmatic patients, the number of differentially expressed genes increased from 1912 to 2721 genes comparing cells at baseline in submerged growth conditions to fully differentiated air-liquid interface cells. Of note, insulin deprivation of bronchial epithelial cells from healthy controls resulted in a similar loss of epithelial differentiation gene expression signatures as seen in asthmatic cells, including the down-regulation of MUC5AC, EPCAM, FGFR2, NOTCH2 and paralleled by upregulation of PERIOSTIN and SERPINB2. This comprehensive study emphasizes the importance of the biological state of the epithelium in determining the transcriptome, a factor often ignored. On the other hand, despite the caveats, epithelial gene expression signatures (eg, PERIOSTIN and SERPINB2) across different studies[17,18,20,25,26] did associate with asthma and could serve as disease biomarkers.

GENOMIC DYSREGULATION IN ASTHMATIC PATIENTS IN RESPONSE TO HUMAN RHINOVIRUS INFECTION

Endotyping and biomarkers identification in non-type 2 asthma has received less attention than type 2–mediated asthma. Based on Th2-high versus Th2-low molecular signatures,[18,27] the incidence of adult non–type 2 asthma may approximate 30%; but this is deceiving because both types may be involved at different stages of the disease.[28] One of the major triggers of severe asthma exacerbations typically inducing a non-type 2 neutrophilic inflammatory response in the upper airways is human rhinovirus (HRV) infection.[29] Genome-wide transcriptome analyses in airway epithelial cells from a small cohort of asthmatic patients and controls have begun to uncover endotypes associated with HRV infection (rhinovirus [RV]-A16) contributing to asthma.[30] Overall, 10 functional pathways were attributable to HRV infection in vitro independent of disease status, including epithelial cilia movement and morphogenesis, type I and type II interferon responses, and innate immune responses. In addition, an overlap of genes enriched for a previously reported Th2 signature[17,18] was shown.[30] For some genes, differential expression in the vehicle-treated cells from asthmatic patients and controls was already present at baseline, indicating an intrinsic molecular difference between asthmatic and nonasthmatic donors before viral infection. In cells from asthmatic patients, sets of genes associated with viral responses were detected, which were related to inflammatory pathways, epithelial structure and remodeling, and cilia assembly and function (eg, CCL5, CXCL10, CX3CL1, MUC5AC, and CDHR3). The investigators concluded that airway epithelial cells derived from asthmatic patients have fundamental structural differences at baseline in the absence of infection, which are further amplified in response to HRV infection. However, cytokine data were not consistent.

To more directly assess the effects on global gene expression patterns in responses to HRV in the host, nasal epithelial cells from adult asthmatic patients and healthy controls were obtained before in vivo inoculation with HRV (RV-A16) as well as at different time points after viral inoculation.[31] Overall changes in the transcriptome were apparent at baseline, during infection, and during the onset of convalescence/repair between both groups. At baseline (7 days before inoculation), 57 genes were differentially expressed between asthmatic patients and controls with lower levels of gene expression of viral replication inhibitors in individuals with asthma together with increased mRNA levels for genes involved in inflammation. In asthmatic patients, a much larger set of genes (n = 1329) was significantly altered from baseline to 36 hours after inoculation. These large gene expression changes were not seen in the control group. An increase in *IL-10* signaling was restricted to healthy individuals without a history of asthma, which may have contributed to a protective effect in these individuals. The investigators suggested that the upregulation of *SPINK5* only in the control group during the convalescence/repair phase identified the potential relevance of this protease inhibitor in the recovery phase.

The effectiveness of whole transcriptome analyses to classify differential responsiveness to clinically relevant stimuli, such as HRV, was used to predict the exacerbation risk in asthmatic children.[32] Biological process pathways were built using a training set based on global expression in peripheral blood mononuclear cells (PBMC) from healthy controls subjected to in vitro exposure to HRV. These classifications were then used to predict exacerbations in asthmatic children[33,34] dependent on gene expression changes in PBMCs before and after virus exposure.[32] Although the classifier was based on healthy controls, asthmatic patients were categorized with a 70% accuracy at low (no exacerbation) or high risk (recurrent exacerbation) to experience an exacerbation. It remains to be confirmed if gene expression in PBMCs reflect mechanistic changes in the lung. However, this minimally invasive procedure showed that developing unbiased genomic profiles combined with a clinically relevant environmental risk assessment can provide a tool to predict exacerbations in asthmatic children.

WHOLE TRANSCRIPTOME ANALYSES AS A MEANS TO PREDICT THE RESPONSE TO CORTICOSTEROID IN ASTHMATIC PATIENTS

The ability to analyze expression levels of thousands of genes at the same time has advanced the identification for molecular mechanisms involved in disease pathobiology, enabled the prediction of asthma exacerbation risk, and aided in defining biomarkers for drug responses in asthmatic patients. To delineate key molecules as predictors, the transcriptome of primary airway smooth muscle cells was studied in response to dexamethasone in a controlled in vitro environment.[35] Overall, 316 genes were altered after dexamethasone exposure, including well-known (*DUSP1, KLF15, PER1, TSC22D3*) and less obvious glucocorticoid-responsive genes (C7, CCDC69, CRISPLD2). *CRISPLD2* was selected for further functional analyses, as single nucleotide polymorphisms in *CRISPLD2* were nominally associated in a genome-wide study for ICS resistance and bronchodilator response. Its role as a potential modulator in the antiinflammatory response to glucocorticoid was further validated after *CRISPLD2* knock-down, which led to an increase in the production of the proinflammatory cytokines IL-6 and IL-8 after stimulation with IL-1β.

Analyzing PBMCs in 2 independent cohorts of steroid-sensitive and steroid-resistant asthmatics, 15 genes separated the response to ICS treatment with a suggested 84% accuracy.[36] Among the identified candidates predicting the clinical response to ICS were NF-κB, *STAT4*, and *IL-4R*, genes associated with asthma pathogenesis.[37–41] A more recent study following whole transcriptome analyses in induced sputum from asthmatic patients distinguished the 4 clinical asthma phenotypes (eosinophilic, non-eosinophilic, pauci-granulocytic or neutrophilic) from healthy controls based on differential expression of 6 key genes (*CLC, CPA3, DNASE1L3, IL-1B, ALPL,* and *CXCR2*) with an area under the curve ranging from 85.7 to 92.6.[42] When changes in expression levels were compared before and after ICS treatment, each of these candidate genes was affected in patients with eosinophilic asthma, strengthening their potential as a useful diagnostic and predictive tool in asthma management.

A similar approach was taken in a small cohort of atopic asthmatic subjects versus atopic and nonatopic controls.[43,44] Endobronchial biopsies were taken before and after 14 days of oral prednisolone or placebo. Each set of subjects was distinguishable through specific gene signatures in bronchial biopsies. In the asthmatic subjects, significant changes in global expression levels were found for 15 genes enriched for 3 pathways in contrast to the placebo group which were associated with cellular growth, proliferation, and development. After the 14-day treatment of oral prednisolone, increased *FAM129A* and *SYNPO2* gene expression was observed which correlated with reduced airway hyperresponsiveness.

Such studies lend support to the relevance of unbiased transcriptional approaches to delineate gene expression profiles that are related to treatment responses. As the number of studies and subjects enrolled are relatively small, further work will be necessary to validate these early findings and explore mechanistic differences in larger cohorts.

SUMMARY

This review selectively summarizes some of the latest developments linking transcriptional biomarkers, endotyping, and clinically relevant asthma outcomes. Distinct transcriptomic profiles have defined complex molecular tissue-specific pathways involved in disease pathogenesis, which may have potential as therapeutic targets. To date, expression of *PERIOSTIN* and *SERPINB2* in epithelial cells appears as the most consistent genetic markers identified across multiple studies.[17,18,20,25,26] Classification of asthmatic patients based on molecular endotypes in addition to traditional clinical parameters will be needed to better assess the heterogeneity of asthma as well as guide personalized interventions to improve outcomes. Although perhaps less vital in the group of patients with steroid-responsive mild-moderate asthma, a molecular approach will be essential in asthmatic patients who fail to respond to CS if we are to intervene in appropriate ways. An important caveat in most of these studies is that they were focused on patients with type 2-high immune responses and were not performed in a longitudinal manner. The best way to study specific interventions with the rapidly increasing number of new biologicals or supplements[45–48] will require more rigid selection criteria for patient entry, in part driven by the dysregulation of distinct pathophysiologic mechanisms, and analyses at more than a single time point.

To improve the effectiveness and applicability of molecular endotyping and biomarker identification, investigations will need to be developed in well-characterized populations with sufficient sample power. As asthma is not a single disease and pathobiology may vary over time, sampling of different immune/inflammatory-relevant cells and tissues from the same patient at multiple time points to monitor longitudinal contributions to disease pathogenesis is needed to address the multifactorial subtypes of asthma. Adding to the complexity are findings that regulatory regions of genes may not be actively transcribed until an appropriate environmental signal is received. It is essential to couple transcriptomic analyses at a steady state as well as after activation to identify genes that truly control expression and to track their stability and/or plasticity over time. Finally, identification of transcriptomic changes mediated through specific genes and/or pathways will only become relevant when the findings are directly coupled to functional outcomes of asthma. This endeavor can only be accomplished by forming consortia using comparable definitions of asthma and disease control, selected target tissues, and uniform analyses of molecular events across studied populations.

ACKNOWLEDGMENTS

The authors would like to thank the National Institutes of Health (grant number AI-77609 and HL-36577), the Eugene F. and Easton M. Crawford Charitable Lead Unitrust, and the Joanne Siegel Fund for their continued support.

REFERENCES

1. Robinson D, Humbert M, Buhl R, et al. Revisiting type 2-high and type 2-low airway inflammation in asthma: current knowledge and therapeutic implications. Clin Exp Allergy 2017;47(2):161–75.

2. Smith AD, Cowan JO, Brassett KP, et al. Use of exhaled nitric oxide measurements to guide treatment in chronic asthma. N Engl J Med 2005;352(21):2163–73.

3. Johansson MW, Evans MD, Crisafi GM, et al. Serum periostin is associated with type-2 immunity in severe asthma. J Allergy Clin Immunol 2016;137(6):1904–7.e2.

4. James A, Janson C, Malinovschi A, et al. Serum periostin relates to type-2 inflammation and lung function in asthma: Data from the large population-based cohort Swedish GA(2)LEN. Allergy 2017;72(11):1753–60.

5. Schleich FN, Manise M, Sele J, et al. Distribution of sputum cellular phenotype in a large asthma cohort: predicting factors for eosinophilic vs neutrophilic inflammation. BMC Pulm Med 2013;13:11.

6. Simpson JL, Scott R, Boyle MJ, et al. Inflammatory subtypes in asthma: assessment and identification using induced sputum. Respirology 2006;11(1):54–61.

7. Chang HS, Lee TH, Jun JA, et al. Neutrophilic inflammation in asthma: mechanisms and therapeutic considerations. Expert Rev Respir Med 2017;11(1):29–40.

8. Green RH, Brightling CE, Woltmann G, et al. Analysis of induced sputum in adults with asthma: identification of subgroup with isolated sputum neutrophilia and poor response to inhaled corticosteroids. Thorax 2002;57(10):875–9.

9. Yan X, Chu JH, Gomez J, et al. Noninvasive analysis of the sputum transcriptome discriminates clinical phenotypes of asthma. Am J Respir Crit Care Med 2015;191(10):1116–25.

10. Shaw DE, Sousa AR, Fowler SJ, et al. Clinical and inflammatory characteristics of the European U-BIOPRED adult severe asthma cohort. Eur Respir J 2015;46(5):1308–21.

11. Rossios C, Pavlidis S, Hoda U, et al. Sputum transcriptomics reveal upregulation of IL-1 receptor family members in patients with severe asthma. J Allergy Clin Immunol 2018;141(2):560–70.

12. Silkoff PE, Strambu I, Laviolette M, et al. Asthma characteristics and biomarkers from the Airways Disease Endotyping for Personalized Therapeutics (ADEPT) longitudinal profiling study. Respir Res 2015;16:142.

13. Peters MC, Mekonnen ZK, Yuan S, et al. Measures of gene expression in sputum cells can identify Th2-high and Th2-low subtypes of asthma. J Allergy Clin Immunol 2014;133(2):388–94.

14. Kuo CS, Pavlidis S, Loza M, et al. T-helper cell type 2 (Th2) and non-Th2 molecular phenotypes of asthma using sputum transcriptomics in U-BIOPRED. Eur Respir J 2017;49(2) [pii:1602135].

15. Hackett TL, Knight DA. The role of epithelial injury and repair in the origins of asthma. Curr Opin Allergy Clin Immunol 2007;7(1):63–8.

16. Kicic A, Hallstrand TS, Sutanto EN, et al. Decreased fibronectin production significantly contributes to dysregulated repair of asthmatic epithelium. Am J Respir Crit Care Med 2010;181(9):889–98.

17. Woodruff PG, Boushey HA, Dolganov GM, et al. Genome-wide profiling identifies epithelial cell genes associated with asthma and with treatment response to corticosteroids. Proc Natl Acad Sci U S A 2007;104(40):15858–63.

18. Woodruff PG, Modrek B, Choy DF, et al. T-helper type 2-driven inflammation defines major subphenotypes of asthma. Am J Respir Crit Care Med 2009;180(5): 388–95.

19. Kuo CS, Pavlidis S, Loza M, et al. A transcriptome-driven analysis of epithelial brushings and bronchial biopsies to define asthma phenotypes in U-BIOPRED. Am J Respir Crit Care Med 2017;195(4):443–55.

20. Poole A, Urbanek C, Eng C, et al. Dissecting childhood asthma with nasal transcriptomics distinguishes subphenotypes of disease. J Allergy Clin Immunol 2014;133(3):670–8.e2.

21. Chung EH, Jia Y, Ohnishi H, et al. Leukotriene B4 receptor 1 is differentially expressed on peripheral T cells of steroid-sensitive and -resistant asthmatics. Ann Allergy Asthma Immunol 2014;112(3):211–216 e1.

22. Ohnishi H, Miyahara N, Dakhama A, et al. Corticosteroids enhance CD8$^+$ T cell-mediated airway hyperresponsiveness and allergic inflammation by upregulating leukotriene B4 receptor 1. J Allergy Clin Immunol 2008;121(4):864–71.e4.

23. Jia Y, Domenico J, Takeda K, et al. Steroidogenic enzyme Cyp11a1 regulates type-2 CD8$^+$ T cell skewing in allergic lung disease. Proc Natl Acad Sci U S A 2013;110(20):8152–7.

24. Jia Y, Takeda K, Han J, et al. Stepwise epigenetic and phenotypic alterations poise CD8$^+$ T cells to mediate airway hyperresponsiveness and inflammation. J Immunol 2013;190(8):4056–65.

25. Singhania A, Wallington JC, Smith CG, et al. Multitissue transcriptomics delineates the diversity of airway T cell functions in asthma. Am J Respir Cell Mol Biol 2018;58(2):261–70.

26. Loffredo LF, Abdala-Valencia H, Anekalla KR, et al. Beyond epithelial-to-mesenchymal transition: common suppression of differentiation programs underlies epithelial barrier dysfunction in mild, moderate, and severe asthma. Allergy 2017;72(12):1988–2004.

27. Baines KJ, Simpson JL, Wood LG, et al. Transcriptional phenotypes of asthma defined by gene expression profiling of induced sputum samples. J Allergy Clin Immunol 2011;127(1):153–60, 160.e1–9.

28. Ray A, Raundhal M, Oriss TB, et al. Current concepts of severe asthma. J Clin Invest 2016;126(7):2394–403.

29. Gavala ML, Bertics PJ, Gern JE. Rhinoviruses, allergic inflammation, and asthma. Immunol Rev 2011;242(1):69–90.

30. Bai J, Smock SL, Jackson GR Jr, et al. Phenotypic responses of differentiated asthmatic human airway epithelial cultures to rhinovirus. PLoS One 2015;10(2): e0118286.

31. Heymann PW, Nguyen HT, Steinke JW, et al. Rhinovirus infection results in stronger and more persistent genomic dysregulation: evidence for altered innate immune response in asthmatics at baseline, early in infection, and during convalescence. PLoS One 2017;12(5):e0178096.

32. Gardeux V, Berghout J, Achour I, et al. A genome-by-environment interaction classifier for precision medicine: personal transcriptome response to rhinovirus identifies children prone to asthma exacerbations. J Am Med Inform Assoc 2017;24(6):1116–26.

33. Lemanske RF Jr, Mauger DT, Sorkness CA, et al. Step-up therapy for children with uncontrolled asthma receiving inhaled corticosteroids. N Engl J Med 2010; 362(11):975–85.

34. Martinez FD, Chinchilli VM, Morgan WJ, et al. Use of beclomethasone dipropionate as rescue treatment for children with mild persistent asthma (TREXA): a

randomised, double-blind, placebo-controlled trial. Lancet 2011;377(9766): 650–7.

35. Himes BE, Jiang X, Wagner P, et al. RNA-Seq transcriptome profiling identifies *CRISPLD2* as a glucocorticoid responsive gene that modulates cytokine function in airway smooth muscle cells. PLoS One 2014;9(6):e99625.

36. Hakonarson H, Bjornsdottir US, Halapi E, et al. Profiling of genes expressed in peripheral blood mononuclear cells predicts glucocorticoid sensitivity in asthma patients. Proc Natl Acad Sci U S A 2005;102(41):14789–94.

37. Schuliga M. NF-kappaB signaling in chronic inflammatory airway disease. Biomolecules 2015;5(3):1266–83.

38. Kumar A, Das S, Agrawal A, et al. Genetic association of key Th1/Th2 pathway candidate genes, IRF2, IL-6, IFNGR2, STAT4 and IL4Rα, with atopic asthma in the Indian population. J Hum Genet 2015;60(8):443–8.

39. Schedel M, Frei R, Bieli C, et al. An IgE-associated polymorphism in STAT6 alters NF-κB binding, STAT6 promoter activity, and mRNA expression. J Allergy Clin Immunol 2009;124(3):583–9, 589.e1–6.

40. Andrews AL, Holloway JW, Holgate ST, et al. IL-4 receptor alpha is an important modulator of IL-4 and IL-13 receptor binding: implications for the development of therapeutic targets. J Immunol 2006;176(12):7456–61.

41. Kabesch M, Schedel M, Carr D, et al. IL-4/IL-13 pathway genetics strongly influence serum IgE levels and childhood asthma. J Allergy Clin Immunol 2006; 117(2):269–74.

42. Baines KJ, Simpson JL, Wood LG, et al. Sputum gene expression signature of 6 biomarkers discriminates asthma inflammatory phenotypes. J Allergy Clin Immunol 2014;133(4):997–1007.

43. Yick CY, Zwinderman AH, Kunst PW, et al. Gene expression profiling of laser microdissected airway smooth muscle tissue in asthma and atopy. Allergy 2014; 69(9):1233–40.

44. Yick CY, Zwinderman AH, Kunst PW, et al. Glucocorticoid-induced changes in gene expression of airway smooth muscle in patients with asthma. Am J Respir Crit Care Med 2013;187(10):1076–84.

45. Haldar P, Brightling CE, Hargadon B, et al. Mepolizumab and exacerbations of refractory eosinophilic asthma. N Engl J Med 2009;360(10):973–84.

46. Humbert M, Busse W, Hanania NA. Controversies and opportunities in severe asthma. Curr Opin Pulm Med 2018;24(1):83–93.

47. Martineau AR, Jolliffe DA, Hooper RL, et al. Vitamin D supplementation to prevent acute respiratory tract infections: systematic review and meta-analysis of individual participant data. BMJ 2017;356:i6583.

48. Vatrella A, Fabozzi I, Calabrese C, et al. Dupilumab: a novel treatment for asthma. J Asthma Allergy 2014;7:123–30.

Exhaled Breath Condensate
An Update

Michael D. Davis, RRT, PhD[a],*, Alison J. Montpetit, RN, PhD[b]

KEYWORDS

- EBC • Exhaled breath condensate • Exhaled breath • Exhaled biomarkers

KEY POINTS

- Exhaled breath condensate (EBC) is a biofluid that contains numerous pulmonary and systemic biomarkers.
- Evidence-based standards of EBC collection, storage, and analysis have been validated, although some controversies related to these topics exist.
- EBC is a valuable tool for researchers and clinicians who seek a noninvasive method to evaluate pulmonary and systemic biomarkers.

Exhaled breath condensate (EBC) is a promising source of biomarkers of lung disease. EBC is not a biomarker, but rather a matrix in which biomarkers may be identified. In that way it is equivalent to blood, sweat, tears, urine, and saliva. There are 3 principal contributors to EBC.[1] First are variable-sized particles or droplets that are aerosolized from the airway lining fluid (ALF)—such particles presumably reflect the fluid itself. Second is distilled water that condenses from gas phase out of the nearly water-saturated exhalate, substantially diluting the aerosolized ALF. Third are water soluble volatiles that are exhaled and absorbed into the condensing breath. Interest lies both in the nonvolatile constituents mostly derived from the ALF particles and in the water-soluble volatile constituents that are found in substantially higher concentrations and are therefore more readily assayed than the nonvolatile compounds.

EBC research and utility has increased substantially over the past 2 decades. The formation of the International Association of Breath Research (IABR) and its Taskforces for the standardization of breath collection and analysis aims to address the

This article is an update of the previously published article on "Exhaled Breath Condensate: An Overview" in the August 2012 issue of the *Immunology and Allergy Clinics of North America*.
Disclosure Statement: M.D. Davis is currently supported by an investigator-initiated award from Mallinckrodt Pharmaceuticals.
[a] Division of Pulmonary Medicine, Children's Hospital of Richmond at VCU, Hermes A. Kontos Medical Sciences Building, Room 215, 1217 East Marshall Street, Richmond, VA 23298, USA;
[b] VCU Medical Center, Department of Emergency Medicine, Box 980401, Richmond, VA 23298-0401, USA
* Corresponding author.
E-mail address: Michael.D.Davis@vcuhealth.org

debates surrounding this emerging field. This review summarizes many of the factors regarding the composition of EBC, its collection, and analysis for the utility of both clinicians and researchers.

SOURCE OF EXHALED BREATH CONDENSATE BIOMARKERS

The nature and source of the exhaled particles/droplets that contribute to the EBC matrix is still largely unknown The aerosolized droplet fraction of EBC has been verified by laser particle counters[2,3]; the presence of these particles serves as the most likely explanation for the presence of nonvolatile constituents in EBC such as cytokines[4] and sodium ion.[5] The mechanism by which these particles form and change during exhalation is not yet confirmed; however, the most widely accepted theory is that small amounts of ALF are liberated from the airway lumen surface by turbulent airflow during exhalation or by recruitment of atelectatic airways sections. Surfactant and surfactant proteins have been found in EBC, which indicates that the alveoli are a source of EBC particles; however, whether these particles aerosolize directly from the alveoli during exhalation or migrate proximally in the airways before aerosolization is unknown.[6]

Of note, the size of particles that are measured exiting the mouth during expiration may be rapidly affected by condensation or evaporation. Size and numerical measurements by laser particle counters therefore reflect the particle size entering the counter, not necessarily the particle size initially generated from the airway lining surface.

PARTICLE SIZE

One 10 micron particle entering a sample of EBC can supply 1,000,000 times the quantity of nonvolatiles to a sample of EBC as one 0.1 micron particle. However, there is skewing of the particle sizes exhaled toward the smaller particles.[3] Overall, the relative contribution to EBC nonvolatile constituents of the different-sized particles remains unknown.

OROPHARYNGEAL CONTRIBUTION TO EXHALED BREATH CONDENSATE

There is no reason to suspect that particles cannot be released from the oral/retro-pharyngeal mucosa into the airstream and potentially contaminate a "pure" lower airway sample. Furthermore, depending in part on the EBC collection equipment, gross or microscopic salivary contamination of EBC can and does occur.[7] Some subjects simply drool during collection, affirming the need for salivary trapping systems to be in place. Measures of salivary amylase are often used to test for the presence of salivary contamination. Most investigators find that no amylase is identified in the great majority of samples, although certainly those using higher sensitivity assays tend to report the presence of measurable amylase in a subset of samples.[7] It is important to mention that the amylase assays used are far from perfect and, similar to all other protein assays in EBC, suffer from some—potentially substantial—amount of false positivity and negativity. Overconfident reliance on any protein assay in EBC not uncommonly has led to mistaken conclusions, and this may be the case for amylase measures as well. Measurable phosphate has been suggested to be reliable indicators of salivary contamination as well.[8] One group concluded that saliva is the source of less than 10% of respiratory droplets.[9]

The ratios among various nonvolatile compounds in EBC have been found to be substantially different than the ratio of compounds in saliva, suggesting a dominant (but not entire) lower airway source of EBC constituents.[9] In oral collections, there is currently no certainty that oral contribution can be completely excluded from the sample. In samples collected by endotracheal tube, there is confidence that the immediate source of volatiles and nonvolatiles is the lower airway and lungs (although aspiration of saliva and gastric fluid can contaminate the lower airway fluid, of course).

DILUTION

The ALF component of EBC is highly diluted by condensing vapor phase water. Estimates of the dilution of ALF particles in EBC range from 20- to 30,000-fold[10]; however, 2000- to 10,000-fold seems to be a generally accepted number.[11] There may be relevant day-to-day and sample-to sample intrasubject variability in dilution, which is further complicated because the assays used for assessment of dilution are themselves a source of variability. As is the case with many biofluids, a gold standard dilution marker for EBC is still sought. Within a given study, it seems worthwhile to attempt to standardize against a relevant additional EBC component, such as the conductivity of a lyophilized sample or ion measurements,[10,12] total protein, or urea measurement.[9] Indeed, in comparison to bronchoalveolar lavage (BAL), it may be easier to obtain a reliable dilution indicator for EBC, because unlike BAL, there is no reasonable mechanism by which collection of EBC significantly alters the ALF.[11]

There are instances when dilution markers are unnecessary for EBC interpretation. One instance is when multiple biomarkers are measured concurrently and their ratios considered. Ratios among interreactive or biologically related biomarkers can be of particular interest and eliminate the need for dilution markers. Examples of such ratios include interferon-gamma ("Th1") to interleukin 4 (IL4) (Th2) ratio,[13,14] nitrite:nitrate (NO_2^- : NO_3^-) ratio,[15] reduced glutathione:oxidized glutathione (GSH:GSSG),[16] and pH (which can be considered a ratio of acids and bases).[17] A second instance in which dilution markers are unnecessary is when there is a confident assay for a substance that serves as an on-off indicator of an abnormality, such as present-not present or plus-minus. Examples might include the presence of *Myobacterium tuberculosis* DNA (by polymerase chain reaction [PCR]), gastric pepsin,[18,19] rhinovirus RNA (by reverse transcription PCR), and anthrax toxin. False positivity in such assays needs to be nil.

LACK OF GOLD STANDARDS OF LUNG DISEASE ASSESSMENT OR DIAGNOSIS WITH WHICH TO COMPARE EXHALED BREATH CONDENSATE MEASUREMENTS

There is still no gold-standard invasive or noninvasive method of determining absolute concentrations of ALF nonvolatile constituents with which EBC can be readily compared. For example, bronchoalveolar lavage is subject to its own dilution concerns and microsampling techniques that draw fluid from the airway wall by capillary action or suction alter the fluid itself. Sputum collection and analysis suffers similarly for 2 reasons: (1) subjects that spontaneously expectorate sputum generally suffer from a disease process, which complicates generation standard values from control subjects, and (2) induction techniques for acquiring sputum from subjects who do not spontaneously expectorate sputum alter the ALF. As a result, there is no consensus as to whether ALF is isotonic, hypo- or hypertonic in comparison to blood. The concentration of sodium ion in the human ALF remains subject to some uncertainty.

The impracticality of invasively collecting samples from healthy lungs additionally limits our knowledge of normal airway fluid components and normal variability. Invasiveness or discomfort of collection drastically limits our ability to study airway components, particularly in healthy subjects not clinically requiring bronchoscopy. These issues underlie the attractiveness of EBC as a research and clinical tool. Importantly, the lack of ability to well access unadulterated ALF using other means should prompt caution if we are overly critical of EBC in light of the above-delineated concerns. In fact, EBC has been used to assess the inflammatory effects of sputum induction that has been shown to increase 2 proinflammatory cytokines, IL6 and tumor necrosis factor alpha.[20] EBC may well be better than other alternatives in assessing the ALF milieu, because it may have fewer drawbacks than other methods.

VALIDATION

EBC is often lumped together with exhaled nitric oxide (eNO) in review articles but is technically far behind eNO from a validation standpoint.[1] One reason for this is that eNO is one biomarker, whereas EBC is a matrix in which hundreds (perhaps thousands) of biomarkers have been identified. A recent search of PubMed reveals 1364 EBC papers, with the first paper published in 1979.[21] Publications involving EBC drastically increased at the turn of the century and have remained steady with an average of 85 publications per year from 2012 to 2017 (**Fig. 1**). These papers cover dozens of diseases/disorders (not including different types of cancers, disease states, and infections) and more than 100 biomarkers. The most common diseases, conditions, and biomarkers are depicted in **Figs. 2** and **3**. In addition, EBC has been evaluated from horses, cows, whales, and dolphins.

COLLECTION OF EXHALED BREATH CONDENSATE

As noted, interest in EBC lies first and foremost with its ease of collection in nearly any setting. The principles of EBC collection are incredibly simple—a subject's breath must simply be directed over a cold surface. Increasing the length of collection time, minute ventilation, and size of the cold surface or decreasing the surface temperature will increase the size of EBC sample collected. EBC can be safely collected orally from spontaneously breathing subjects or from patients undergoing mechanical

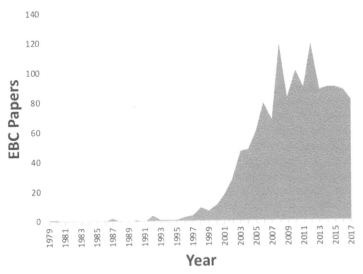

Fig. 1. EBC publications by year in the peer-reviewed literature.

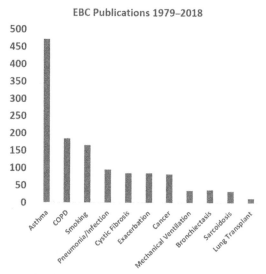

Fig. 2. EBC publications by disease/disorder in the peer-reviewed literature.

ventilation.[22–24] The methods of collection for these settings, while both simple, vary somewhat.

ORAL COLLECTION

It takes as little as one breath to collect EBC, although in research practice, substantially longer collection times are often used to assure sufficient sample is available for

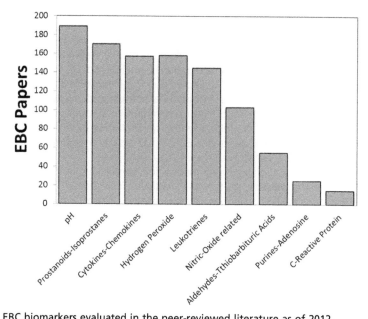

Fig. 3. EBC biomarkers evaluated in the peer-reviewed literature as of 2012.

repeated analysis of multiple biomarkers. Ten minutes of oral tidal breathing yields 1 to 2 mL of sample and is well tolerated. Because modern analytical techniques use smaller sample volumes than was previously required (some as little at 5 μL per analyte), some centers are collecting EBC for shorter durations. At our center, the most common oral EBC collection duration is 10 minutes.

Several options exist for collection of EBC samples from both spontaneously breathing and mechanically ventilated patients (**Table 1**). Multiple custom devices have been used throughout the years, using various cooling techniques, device shapes, materials, and coatings. The components used to create simple home-made systems usually include disposable respiratory adapters, tubing, and ice/dry ice, all of which are generally available in a respiratory or anesthesia clinical setting (and are inexpensive). Commercially available equipment is also available. Certain biomarkers are seemingly best collected under set condensation conditions, but these conditions are markedly different for various biomarkers.[11] Although standardized methods of collection and storage for certain individual biomarkers are developing, there is no expectation that there will ever be a standardized EBC collection procedure that will be uniform for all biomarkers. Therefore, any collection method that satisfies the needs of the user and biomarker is acceptable, but there is not, nor should there be, a one-size-fits-all standardized methodology.

COLLECTION DURING MECHANICAL VENTILATION

Although EBC collection during mechanical ventilation follows the same simple principles listed earlier, there are several considerations specific to this patient population. The length of time needed to collect an adequate sample depends on the device used for collection (see **Table 1**), the patient (ie, higher volumes of EBC are obtained per given period of time in adults vs neonates), and the humidity devices/settings used (if any) during mechanical ventilation.[24] Samples collected from subjects receiving humidified mechanical ventilation will be diluted by the humidified bias flow that travels through the condenser (along with the exhaled breath). Reducing the humidity of the gas delivered to the patient may not be tolerated by the patient and will significantly reduce the amount of EBC sample collected over time but will provide less dilute EBC. Dilution of the sample is less likely to affect the measurement of biomarker ratios than specific biomarkers. Another consideration is that EBC collected orally may have different biomarker ranges than EBC collected during mechanical ventilation, because the upper airway is bypassed by the endotracheal or tracheostomy tube. The authors' group conducted a study of EBC pH pre-/postintubation and it does not change in healthy subjects[25]; however, the relatively low concentration of ammonia (a base) in endotracheally collected EBC allows for EBC pH to be a more sensitive indicator of airway acidification in intubated than nonintubated subjects.

EBC can be collected 2 ways during mechanical ventilation: in-line with the ventilator circuit or at the exhaust port of the ventilator (see **Table 1**). Both methods have pros and cons. In-line collection can be collected closer to the patient (on the expiratory end of the ventilator wye) and is therefore likely to trap larger particles in EBC that may rain out into the ventilator circuit before reaching the exhaust port. Downsides to in-line collection are the need to open the ventilator circuit in order to place and remove the collection device; this requires interrupting. Also, current in-line collection does not allow for analysis of EBC in real-time and, depending on the device, may limit the amount of EBC sample that can be collected (typically <5 mL). Collection at the exhaust port (post ventilator) does not require an interruption of ventilation and can allow for continuous collection EBC and even measurement of EBC pH

Table 1
Current exhaled breath condensate collection systems commonly used

EBC Collection System	Manufacturer	Advantages	Disadvantages
ECoScreen I/II	Carefusion, Europe	Most commonly published EBC collection system. More common in European centers. Optional package for determination of total exhaled volume. Has been used to collect EBC during mechanical ventilation.	Not readily portable. Cleaning between patients may need to be extensive to abide by standard respiratory care practices. Limited ability to control condensation temperature. No longer distributed in the United States.
ECoScreen Turbo	Carefusion, Europe	Lightweight, portable condenser system. Controllable condenser temperature. Disposable collection circuit. Optional package for determination of total exhaled volume.	Few publications. No longer distributed in the United States.
RTube	Respiratory Research, USA	More total EBC collections performed using RTube than other systems. Multiple collections can be performed concurrently. More common in North American centers. Disposable (no cleaning between patients). Portable. Can be prepared for use in a standard freezer, enabling home collection.	Choice and maintenance of set condensing temperature requires optional cooling unit; otherwise condensation temperature is chosen by cooling sleeve preparation temperature and increases during collection.
RTube Vent	Respiratory Research, USA	Can be used in-line with ventilator circuit or at expiratory port. Insignificant resistance regardless of placement in ventilator circuit.	Choice and maintenance of set condensing temperature requires optional cooling unit; otherwise condensation temperature is chosen by cooling sleeve preparation temperature and rises during collection. Few publications (safety data only).
ALFA	Respiratory Research, USA	Has both nondisposable and disposable portions. Controllable collection temperature. Collects EBC continuously throughout the course of ventilation. Gas standardizes and measures EBC pH continuously. Compatible with most ventilators.	Few publications. Complex system, so requires skilled user. Only able to collect EBC at exhaust port of ventilator.

in real-time.[22] Recent technological advances in mechanical ventilation EBC collection methods are stimulating this area of EBC research. Certain mechanical ventilators may alter their function in the presence of an EBC collection system, so it is important for a respiratory therapist or other experienced individual to formally assess how the devices interact.

RANGE OF EXHALED BREATH CONDENSATE BIOMARKERS

Categorization of EBC biomarkers has been done in the past,[11] although it is open to change. There are several potential categorizations, and biomarkers may fall into one or more of the following groups:

Categorization group 1
- Volatile compounds
- Nonvolatile compounds
- Nonvolatile compounds derived from volatile compounds

Categorization group 2
- Very low-molecular-weight compounds
- Low-molecular-weight compounds
- Polypeptides
- Proteins
- Nucleic acids

Miscellaneous differentiation
- Lipid mediators
- Inorganic molecules
- Organic molecules
- Redox-relevant molecules
- pH-relevant molecules
- Cytokines, chemokines

There is no reason to suspect that anything more than a tiny minority of potentially relevant compounds have been reported as of yet. Given a sufficiently sensitive assay, it is likely that any reasonably stable molecule in the ALF can be found in EBC, and more useful EBC biomarker categories will result from new findings.

The most substantive difference among these categories is that between volatile and nonvolatile constituents. As an introductory caveat, it is important to note that some clearly nonvolatile compounds found in EBC may be derivatives of volatiles. For example, nitrate (NO_3^-) and nitrite (NO_2^-)—ionized and therefore not volatile—may arise in EBC in part from a reaction of volatile gaseous nitric oxide (NO) after reaction with oxygen.[26] Chloride ion (Cl^-), another nonvolatile, can be at least in part delivered as the volatile hydrochloric acid (HCl).

Volatiles

Volatiles such as acetic acid, formic acid, and ammonia are found in much higher concentrations in EBC than nonvolatile constituents, and tend, therefore, to be much easier to measure. Volatile biomarkers may be identified in the high micromolar or even low millimolar range, and current state-of-the-art analytical devices are capable of discovering new markers in the nano- and picomolar ranges. Their arrival and concentration in EBC is controlled by entirely different factors than the nonvolatile biomarkers. Indeed, the amount and size of particles formed by turbulence are nearly irrelevant for volatile biomarkers due to the previously mentioned relative dilution of particles in EBC.

However, other factors are important in regard to interpretation of volatile biomarker levels, including water solubility, gas–liquid partition coefficients, temperature of the source fluid (ALF), temperature of the condenser, pH of the source fluid and EBC, and the opportunity to react within (and therefore be captured by) the EBC matrix or collection device itself. An elevated level of formic acid in EBC may not mean more formic acid production in the ALF but rather may indicate a lower pH of the ALF (and therefore enhanced volatility because nonvolatile formate ion is protonated in acidic fluid to form the somewhat volatile species formic acid). Much of the importance of EBC pH as an indicator of ALF pH is because of this feature of volatile acids and bases: acids tend to be volatile from, whereas bases tend to be trapped by, acidity. When EBC pH is lower than normal, more acid and/or less base has been delivered to and captured in the EBC, primarily because more acid and less base has been volatilized from an acidic airway. Although EBC pH does not equal airway pH, an acidic EBC is indeed created from an acidic airway source fluid, so qualitative noninvasive assessments of airway pH deviation become achievable.

Some of the issues so far determined to be relevant to control for when planning to assay volatiles include the following:

1. Condensation temperature that is sufficiently cold to freeze the EBC may diminish the amount of volatiles (which are more readily absorbed into the liquid phase).[25]
2. Frozen storage may protect reactive or unstable compounds, but may also allow sublimation of the volatiles into the airspace above the frozen EBC (unpublished observation, Hunt, 2007). These volatiles will be lost when the storage container is opened, unless efforts are made to thaw and remix the sample before opening.
3. Volatile substances respond differently to sample manipulation. Each substance of interest should be studied well to control for potential effects of collection duration, temperature, storage conditions, and assay system.

Nonvolatiles

Nonvolatile constituents of EBC make up a broad category containing molecules as small as sodium ion (Na+) and as large as immunoglobulins. There are numerous publications in the literature presenting an individual compound that has been found in EBC (relying often on one assay) with levels depending on disease state, with speculations added that the biomarker may be valuable in managing the disease of interest. When attempting to validate a novel EBC biomarker, the authors recommend the following:

1. Confirmation of results of your assay with other assays using different methodology.
2. Assurance that assay controls are performed appropriately and thoroughly.
   - This is perhaps the single most important point for investigators studying EBC. EBC is a highly dilute, low-protein aqueous matrix. If one uses commercially available assay kits for EBC, it is important to assure that the standards used for comparison (standard curve generation) are done in a matrix as similar to that EBC sample as possible. The artifact-producing effect of using improper standards is often called a "matrix effect" and can be substantial in EBC assays.[27] Using proteinaceous standards ("cytokine X in BSA") and attempting to compare to unaltered EBC will likely lead to misleading assay values. One choice is for the EBC sample to be altered so as to be substantially similar to the standards (such as by adding albumin, as the case may be). Because of

inadequate recognition of matrix effect, it is likely that some of the published data are contaminated by artifacts sufficiently to invalidate their conclusions.

○ Also, many, if not most, of the nonvolatile constituents found within EBC are identified by assays pushing their lower limits of accuracy. On the one hand, great care should be taken to assure that the assay is reporting correctly. On the other hand, expectations for assay reproducibility at these low levels cannot be overly high. EBC biomarkers have often been critiqued as suffering from high intrasubject variability and therefore of marginal value. In many cases, however, this variability may greatly result from *assay* variability as opposed to biological or EBC collection system variability. Such assay variability is found for dilution assessment efforts as well, which can mathematically compound the overall nonbiological variability and if not accounted for can lead to incorrect conclusions exaggerating the apparent biological variability or EBC collection system variability.

3. Awareness that the pH of EBC does vary in disease states substantially, with pH values as low as 3.5 and as high as 9.0 reported.[17,28] Because the reactivities and stabilities of many of the other biomarkers of interest are affected by the pH of the fluid in which they are found, and because accuracy of some assays can be affected as well, investigators need to be aware that EBC pH can cause assay artifact as well as loss (or gain) of biomarkers in EBC during storage.

4. Recognition that, in the absence of dilution assessment, different levels of a *single* EBC biomarker in a disease state may be interpreted to represent different levels of the biomarker in the ALF or a different amount/size of particles evolved from an otherwise identical ALF. To reiterate an earlier point, ratios among more than one related biomarker do not require dilution markers to be of more confident value.

A key point is that conscientious assay technique will likely find in EBC any substance of substantially high concentration in the ALF. It is beyond the scope of this article to provide details regarding each of the biomarkers that has been reported in EBC, and the field is advancing with new discoveries weekly.

INTERPRETATION OF EXHALED BREATH CONDENSATE BIOMARKERS

One of the major challenges in interpreting EBC biomarkers is the difficulty in comparing findings across studies. First, despite EBC methodological recommendations set forth by an ATS/ERS task force in 2005, many investigators do not fully describe collection methods.[11] Second, there are multiple areas for variation in biomarker assays:

1. Differences between laboratories or users,
2. Differences between manufacturers or assay kits for the same biomarker, and
3. Differences between kit lot numbers from the same manufacturer.

This makes it difficult to compare biomarker concentrations from one study to another. One recommendation is to analyze biomarker trends in terms of relative change rather than absolute concentration. Third, most biomarkers do not have established normal values or ranges. One method to overcome this deficiency is to describe biomarker variations in the context of the individual subject's baseline where they serve as their own control. Clearly, one of the major needs in EBC research is the establishment of methodological standards and normative values specific to each EBC biomarker. Ongoing attempts by task forces of the IABR aim to provide standardization recommendations and guidelines for EBC utility.

FUTURE OF EXHALED BREATH CONDENSATE RESEARCH

With the formation of the IABR in 2005, the development of the *Journal of Breath Research* in 2007, and the annual Breath Analysis Summits,[29] EBC research is advancing. As EBC research and resulting literature expand, more methodological studies, reviews, and meta-analyses will be conducted in order to fully develop EBC science and adequately assess the clinical relevance of EBC biomarkers. Exhaled biomarkers are ideal for many reasons but primarily because they are safe, noninvasive, can be repeatedly measured, and represent the airway milieu. Exhaled breath may reveal more subtle changes in the airway, although it is yet unknown if exhaled biomarkers will show disease-induced variations earlier than traditional systemic markers (eg, serum/plasma) and/or pulmonary diagnostics (eg, pulmonary function testing, chest radiograph). Because of the array of biomarkers that can be assessed in exhaled breath, ease of collection, and recent advances in technology, exhaled biomarkers have become an exciting field of research despite methodological issues. Development of sensitive tools for monitoring pulmonary diseases could potentially reduce patient burden; increase patient safety during diagnostic testing; aid in earlier diagnosis; and give pulmonary-specific indicators of disease state, impending infection, and/or treatment effects. Exhaled breath research will expand our understanding of pathophysiologic mechanisms underlying pulmonary disease and provide a possible future for development of point-of-care testing. EBC research is an exciting, challenging, and rapidly evolving line of inquiry.

REFERENCES

1. Hunt J. Exhaled breath condensate: an evolving tool for noninvasive evaluation of lung disease. J Allergy Clin Immunol 2002;110(1):28–34.
2. Fairchild CI, Stampfer JF. Particle concentration in exhaled breath. Am Ind Hyg Assoc J 1987;48(11):948–9.
3. Papineni RS, Rosenthal FS. The size distribution of droplets in the exhaled breath of healthy human subjects. J Aerosol Med 1997;10(2):105–16.
4. Tufvesson E, Bjermer L. Methodological improvements for measuring eicosanoids and cytokines in exhaled breath condensate. Respir Med 2006;100(1): 34–8.
5. Zacharasiewicz A, Wilson N, Lex C, et al. Repeatability of sodium and chloride in exhaled breath condensates. Pediatr Pulmonol 2004;37(3):273–5.
6. Sidorenko GI, Zborovskii EI, Levina DI. Surface-active properties of the exhaled air condensate (a new method of studying lung function). Ter Arkh 1980;52(3): 65–8 [in Russian].
7. Gaber F, Acevedo F, Delin I, et al. Saliva is one likely source of leukotriene B4 in exhaled breath condensate. Eur Respir J 2006;28(6):1229–35.
8. Griese M, Noss J, Bredow Cv C. Protein pattern of exhaled breath condensate and saliva. Proteomics 2002;2(6):690–6.
9. Effros RM, Peterson B, Casaburi R, et al. Epithelial lining fluid solute concentrations in chronic obstructive lung disease patients and normal subjects. J Appl Physiol (1985) 2005;99(4):1286–92.
10. Effros RM, Hoagland KW, Bosbous M, et al. Dilution of respiratory solutes in exhaled condensates. Am J Respir Crit Care Med 2002;165(5):663–9.
11. Horvath I, Hunt J, Barnes PJ, et al. Exhaled breath condensate: methodological recommendations and unresolved questions. Eur Respir J 2005;26(3):523–48.

12. Effros RM, Biller J, Foss B, et al. A simple method for estimating respiratory solute dilution in exhaled breath condensates. Am J Respir Crit Care Med 2003;168(12): 1500–5.
13. Shahid SK, Kharitonov SA, Wilson NM, et al. Increased interleukin-4 and decreased interferon-gamma in exhaled breath condensate of children with asthma. Am J Respir Crit Care Med 2002;165(9):1290–3.
14. Robroeks CM, Jobsis Q, Damoiseaux JG, et al. Cytokines in exhaled breath condensate of children with asthma and cystic fibrosis. Ann Allergy Asthma Immunol 2006;96(2):349–55.
15. Nguyen TA, Woo-Park J, Hess M, et al. Assaying all of the nitrogen oxides in breath modifies the interpretation of exhaled nitric oxide. Vascul Pharmacol 2005;43(6):379–84.
16. Yeh MY, Burnham EL, Moss M, et al. Non-invasive evaluation of pulmonary glutathione in the exhaled breath condensate of otherwise healthy alcoholics. Respir Med 2008;102(2):248–55.
17. Paget-Brown AO, Ngamtrakulpanit L, Smith A, et al. Normative data for pH of exhaled breath condensate. Chest 2006;129(2):426–30.
18. Samuels TL, Johnston N. Pepsin as a marker of extraesophageal reflux. Ann Otol Rhinol Laryngol 2010;119(3):203–8.
19. Timms C, Thomas PS, Yates DH. Detection of gastro-oesophageal reflux disease (GORD) in patients with obstructive lung disease using exhaled breath profiling. J Breath Res 2012;6(1):016003.
20. Carpagnano GE, Foschino Barbaro MP, Cagnazzo M, et al. Use of exhaled breath condensate in the study of airway inflammation after hypertonic saline solution challenge. Chest 2005;128(5):3159–66.
21. Larson TV, Covert DS, Frank R. A method for continuous measurement of ammonia in respiratory airways. J Appl Physiol 1979;46(3):603–7.
22. Walsh BK, Mackey DJ, Pajewski T, et al. Exhaled-breath condensate pH can be safely and continuously monitored in mechanically ventilated patients. Respir Care 2006;51(10):1125–31.
23. Muller WG, Morini F, Eaton S, et al. Safety and feasibility of exhaled breath condensate collection in ventilated infants and children. Eur Respir J 2006; 28(3):479–85.
24. Carter SR, Davis CS, Kovacs EJ. Exhaled breath condensate collection in the mechanically ventilated patient. Respir Med 2012;106(5):601–13.
25. Vaughan J, Ngamtrakulpanit L, Pajewski TN, et al. Exhaled breath condensate pH is a robust and reproducible assay of airway acidity. Eur Respir J 2003;22(6): 889–94.
26. Hunt J, Byrns RE, Ignarro LJ, et al. Condensed expirate nitrite as a home marker for acute asthma [letter]. Lancet 1995;346(8984):1235–6.
27. Hom S, Walsh B, Hunt J. Matrix effect in exhaled breath condensate interferon-gamma immunoassay. J Breath Res 2008;2(4):041001.
28. Nicolaou NC, Lowe LA, Murray CS, et al. Exhaled breath condensate pH and childhood asthma: unselected birth cohort study. Am J Respir Crit Care Med 2006;174(3):254–9.
29. Corradi M, Mutti A. News from the breath analysis summit 2011. J Breath Res 2012;6(2):020201.

Biomarkers in Chronic Rhinosinusitis with Nasal Polyps

Alan D. Workman, MD, MTR[a], Michael A. Kohanski, MD, PhD[a],
Noam A. Cohen, MD, PhD[a,b,c],*

KEYWORDS

- Chronic rhinosinusitis • Biomarkers • Polyps • Microbiome • Genetics

KEY POINTS

- Chronic rhinosinusitis is a complex disease that exists along the inflammatory spectrum between types 1 and 2 inflammation.
- The classic phenotypic differentiation of chronic rhinosinusitis based on the presence or absence of inflammatory polyps remains one of the best differentiators of response to therapy.
- Biologics for the treatment of atopic disease and asthma, and perhaps a new look at topical therapies for sinusitis, have placed renewed emphasis on understanding the pathophysiology of inflammatory sinus polyp pathogenesis.
- Identification of key markers of polyposis will allow for better stratification of inflammatory polyp disease endotypes to objectively identify tailored medical therapies and track response to medical and surgical treatment.

INTRODUCTION

Chronic rhinosinusitis (CRS) is a prevalent and heterogeneous disease associated with a high degree of morbidity. Although there exist specific conditions for diagnosis, it has been increasingly appreciated that CRS exists as a spectrum of clinical conditions with distinct pathophysiology and presentation.[1] Targeted biologics for treating asthma are now being used for CRS with nasal polyps (CRSwNP), which has

[a] Department of Otorhinolaryngology–Head and Neck Surgery, Division of Rhinology, University of Pennsylvania, Perelman School of Medicine, 3400 Spruce Street, Philadelphia, PA 19104, USA; [b] Philadelphia Veterans Affairs Medical Center, 3900 Woodland Avenue, Philadelphia, PA 19104, USA; [c] Monell Chemical Senses Center, 3500 Market Street, Philadelphia, PA 19104, USA
* Corresponding author. Division of Rhinology, Department of Otorhinolaryngology–Head and Neck Surgery, University of Pennsylvania Medical Center, 5th Floor Ravdin Building, 3400 Spruce Street, Philadelphia, PA 19104.
E-mail address: Noam.Cohen@uphs.upenn.edu

Immunol Allergy Clin N Am 38 (2018) 679–692
https://doi.org/10.1016/j.iac.2018.06.006
0889-8561/18/Published by Elsevier Inc.
immunology.theclinics.com

predicated the need for improved classification and diagnosis of different presentations of the disease in an effort to improve therapeutic efficacy.

Traditionally, a dichotomous classification system has been used to describe CRS based on the presence or absence of nasal polyps. CRSwNP represents a subset of those with CRS,[2] and CRSwNP is often associated with more severe sinonasal symptoms and asthma. The division of CRS by polyp status was initially supported at the cellular level, with CRS without nasal polyps (CRSsNP) thought to be characterized by a T-helper type 1 (T_H1)-predominant inflammatory pattern and CRSwNP characterized by a T-helper type 2 (T_H2)-predominant inflammatory pattern. However, recent work has demonstrated that CRS may be better evaluated as a continuum of inflammatory processes, with variable and nonmutually exclusive immunologic markers. This complexity can potentially be captured with endotype or cluster classification based on consistent pathologic mechanisms that may not be evident at the level of phenotypic observation. Endotypes are often defined by the presence or absence of one or more biomarkers, and the use of biomarkers can be helpful in achieving accurate diagnosis, evaluating optimal therapeutic strategy, and determining patient prognosis.

Chronic Rhinosinusitis with Nasal Polyps Pathophysiology

Inflammatory sinonasal polyps manifest bilaterally from the ethmoid sinuses and can often present with hyposmia and/or nasal obstruction as major symptoms (**Figs. 1 and 2**). It is thought that nasal polyp growth is present in 1% to 4% of the US population.[3] As stated, T_H2 inflammation often predominates and is associated with elevated levels of eosinophils and type 2 inflammatory cytokines including IL-4, IL-5, and IL-13.[4] Asthma is frequently a comorbid condition in patients with CRSwNP, affecting 20% to 60% of diseased individuals.[5] An additional hallmark of CRSwNP is the loss of healthy barrier function in sinonasal epithelial cells. There is generally increased permeability, decreased epithelial resistance, and a high degree of tissue remodeling observed[6] in cells harvested from patients with CRSwNP compared with cells from CRSsNP patients and control individuals. This loss of barrier function is reflective of a general inflammatory process, but it is unclear whether the epithelial cells are inherently abnormal or if the state is induced.[7] Treatment for CRS is most frequently glucocorticoid based, but response is quite variable in patients with nasal polyps and the side effects from oral steroids limits their long-term efficacy in the treatment of this disease. Hamilos and colleagues[8] demonstrated an inverse relationship between glucocorticoid receptor-β expression in nasal polyp tissue and steroid efficacy, and another study showed that neutrophil accumulation in nasal polyp tissue is also related to corticosteroid insensitivity.[9] Some individuals exhibit a very high level of resistance to steroid therapy, and this underscores the need for therapeutics targeted toward non–steroid-responsive pathophysiologic mechanisms involved in sinus polyp formation.

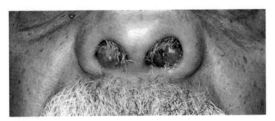

Fig. 1. Visible nasal polyps on external nares examination.

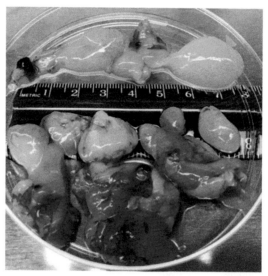

Fig. 2. Removed nasal polyps after functional endoscopic sinus surgery.

BIOMARKERS AND THERAPEUTICS IN CHRONIC RHINOSINUSITIS WITH NASAL POLYPS

An ideal biomarker is easy to obtain and has a high sensitivity and specificity for the disease or disease subtype in question. The most frequently used mediums to obtain CRS biomarkers are peripheral blood, nasal secretions, tissue biopsies from the sinuses, and nasally exhaled breath. A peripheral blood draw is significantly easier to obtain than a nasal biopsy, and requires less time, expertise, and expense. However, peripheral blood may not always reflect local nasal inflammatory processes and is often a poor proxy for the nasal microenvironment. Nasal lavage is more useful in many situations, but several studies have demonstrated a somewhat inconsistent correlation between cytokines and proteins in nasal secretions and those in the tissue itself.[4] Much of this is likely due to geographic variability in inflammatory microenvironments in the sinonasal environment. Many CRS biomarkers have been preliminarily evaluated in recent years (**Table 1**), with most of the literature expanding on proof-of-concept studies of markers that have been evaluated in related diseases, including asthma, environmental aeroallergens, and atopic dermatitis.

Eosinophilia and IgE

Classically, CRSwNP is an eosinophilic disease and CRSsNP is generally noneosinophilic. However, there are many random and regional exceptions, with up to 50% of patients with CRSwNP in East Asia presenting without eosinophilic inflammation.[10] Wang and associates[11] further showed that 20% to 75% of nasal polyp specimens can be noneosinophilic, contrasted with tissue obtained from CRSsNP patients that can show very high eosinophilia in a minority of cases. Although this substantial overlap prohibits the use of eosinophilia as a definitive marker for polyp disease, eosinophilia itself can be a predictive tool. Eosinophilic nasal polyps are associated with increased objective and subjective disease severity, as well as an increased risk of recurrence of disease after sinus surgery.[12] Conversely, eosinophilic polyps are generally more glucocorticoid responsive than their noneosinophilic counterparts.[9]

Table 1
List of current biomarkers

Biomarker	Source Medium	Targeted Therapy
Eosinophilia	Tissue, peripheral blood	
IgE	Tissue	Omalizumab
Cytokines		
IL-4	Tissue	Dupilumab
IL-5	Tissue	Mepolizumab, reslizumab
IL-13	Tissue	Dupilumab
IL-25	Tissue	
IL-33	Tissue	
Thymic stromal lymphoprotein	Tissue	
Periostin	Tissue, nasal secretions	
P-glycoprotein	Tissue, nasal secretions	Verapamil
CXCL-12/CXCL-13	Tissue	
Type 2 innate lymphoid cells	Tissue	
IgG and IgA autoantibodies	Tissue	
Nitric oxide	Exhaled breath	
Bitter and sweet taste receptors	Tissue, genotype, taste test	
Microbiome	Nasal secretions	
IgE antibody to Staphylococcus aureus enterotoxin	Tissue	
Matrix metalloproteinases	Tissue, nasal secretions	Doxycycline
Oncostatin M	Tissue	

Classification of an eosinophilic-rich environment is most often achieved using tissue microscopy, with different groups establishing optimal cutoffs for grading levels of eosinophilia. Kountakis and colleagues[13] established a cutoff point of greater than 5 eosinophils per high power field, whereas Soler and colleagues[14] had a higher cutoff of 10 eosinophils per high-power field based on a measurement of quality of life improvement after surgery. Importantly, degree of tissue eosinophilia is extremely difficult to determine based on clinical symptoms, and it cannot be predicted by SNOT-22 scores or the concomitant presence of asthma or aspirin-exacerbated respiratory disease.[15] Whereas many studies establish that it is possible to identify a cohort of patients with noneosinophilic nasal polyp and a cohort of hypereosinophilic nasal polyp patients, most patients fall along an expression continuum that makes grouping solely on eosinophilia difficult.[15] Further experiments have used blood eosinophilia to predict disease relapse after surgery, but this is complicated by the fact that blood eosinophilia is not definitively correlated with that in tissue.[16]

IgE, an inducer of eosinophilia, has also been investigated as a biomarker for CRS phenotyping and treatment. Patients with CRS frequently express high levels of serum and local IgE, in addition to allergic sensitization to bacterial antigens.[17] Specifically, *Staphylococcus aureus* enterotoxins can serve as both conventional and superantigens to activate basophil degranulation in those with CRSwNP.[18] High local IgE in tissue itself was also predictive of recurrence requiring repeat surgical intervention.[19] The anti-IgE therapeutic omalizumab was also tested in patients with CRSwNP to see if it could reduce polyp burden and lead to symptomatic improvement. Omalizumab reduced nasal polyp size and improved sinus computed tomography scores in patients with CRSwNP, but decreases in local nasal mucosal inflammation were not unequivocally observed.[20]

Cytokines

Cytokine profiles are perhaps the most currently investigated and initially promising biomarkers for CRS phenotyping and therapeutic targets. The classic characterization of CRSsNP is with a T_H1 or T_H17 phenotype with prominent neutrophilia, expressing transforming growth factor-β, type I interferons, and IL-6, IL-8, or IL-17. This is contrasted with the characterization of CRSwNP as a T_H2 microenvironment with increased expression of thymic stromal lymphoprotein and type 2 inflammatory cells, such as type 2 innate lymphoid cells, which produce IL-4, IL-5, IL-13, IL-25, and/or IL-33. Type 2 innate lymphoid cells play a role in T- and B-cell activation, and activated epithelial cells contribute to leaky barriers as they apoptose.[1] Both IL-4 and IL-13 induce local IgE production and stimulate mucus secretion, whereas IL-5 induces eosinophilia through the recruitment, activation, and survival of eosinophils.[1] IL-13 affects epithelial differentiation resulting in decreased ciliation and goblet cell metaplasia, further contributing to a leaky epithelial barrier of sinonasal epithelial cells.[21] IL-13 also increases hyperreactivity of the airway and causes subepithelial fibrosis. More recently, studies show that IL-25 seems to be involved in the IL-13 regulatory cascade, with IL-25 stimulation inducing IL-13–dependent changes in an asthma mouse model.[22]

Cytokine signatures are extremely valuable in determining T_H classification and are more specific than eosinophilia or even the presence of nasal polyps themselves, even though both are more common in T_H2 high states.[23] The T_H1 and T_H2 dichotomy is useful but also an oversimplification as a proxy for nasal polyp status. Eighty-five percent of nasal polyps do have high concentrations of IL-5, but there is intermittent concomitant expression of IL-17 and interferon-γ that is more characteristic of a T_H1 process.[11] The subset of patients with IL-5–enriched nasal polyps has an increased percentage of asthma and revision surgery patients.[24] The presence of IL-5 may be defining for a specific endotype of CRSwNP individuals with more severe disease. IL-25, IL-33, and thymic stromal lymphoprotein are also epithelial-derived cytokines that are important in the pathogenesis of CRSwNP and asthma, and may be important biomarkers for CRSwNP. IL-25 expression is upregulated in CRSwNP tissue,[25] is associated with elevated eosinophil counts and increased severity in computed tomography scoring parameters,[26] and can potentially serve as a sensitive biomarker.[27] IL-33 participates in less well-defined pathways, but also plays a role in T_H2 inflammation. IL-33 expression levels are increased specifically in patients with CRSwNP with severe and recalcitrant disease.[28]

Many anticytokine agents are currently in production and development as asthma treatments, and it is a logical extension that they may have a potential role in treating T_H2 inflammation in CRS. It has been well-demonstrated that asthmatic patients with a T_H2 phenotype with eosinophilia derive benefit from IL-5 antagonists.[29] In fact, nasal polyps were a good biomarker for predicting anti–IL-5 response in these studies, owing to the relationship of nasal polyps with a T_H2-skewed state. Antibodies to IL-5 already are approved for refractory asthma, and an anti–IL-5 receptor antibody will be available in a short time. Initial trials of IL-5 antagonism with mepolizumab and reslizumab in CRSwNP demonstrated a reduction in nasal polyp size and reduced necessity for revision surgeries.[30,31] However, these trials have not definitively shown improved nasal symptom sores, and careful patient selection may be critical for derivation of benefit. An IL-5–enriched endotype seems to be necessary to predict efficacy, because eosinophil markers themselves were not predictive of mepolizumab response magnitudes.[32]

Dupilumab is an anti–IL-4 receptor antibody that blocks the actions of both IL-4 and IL-13 that is currently used in atopic dermatitis and has shown efficacy in treating asthmatics with an elevated type 2 inflammatory response.[33] Just as with anti–IL-5 treatments, dupilumab also improves several outcomes in patients with CRSwNP from clinical, endoscopic, and radiologic standpoints.[34] Nasal polyps decrease in size and sinus computed tomography scores are less severe after treatment, although objective sinus symptomatology measures and smell tests also show improvement in patients with a confirmed T_H2/eosinophil endotype.[34] Again, the effectiveness of these treatments is predicated on a well-defined and compatible inflammatory signature, so appropriate patient selection for therapy is important.[35] Murine studies also show promise for IL-25 blockade, because polypoid lesions are reduced and edematous inflammation is decreased at the cellular and mucosal level.[36] These novel cytokine pathways are very promising targets for CRSwNP therapies in the coming years, and diagnostic tools incorporating these cytokines will be concomitantly necessary for patient selection. Some studies have purported that the cytokines in nasal secretions correlate with tissue levels to a degree that allows for alternative evaluation, and can be useful when assessment of structural and cellular patterns of expression are not necessary.[37] Longitudinal tracking of biomarkers will also be important to objectively measure therapeutic efficacy, because the cost of biologics is currently prohibitive for CRS. The current cost of dupilumab treatment for nasal polyps is greater than treating the condition with surgery every 6 months for the duration of symptomatology.[38]

Periostin

Periostin is an extracellular protein that is secreted in response to IL-4 and IL-13 and it plays a role in airway subepithelial fibrosis through interactions with integrin molecules involved in tissue remodeling.[39] Additionally, it participates in eosinophil recruitment and activation cascades as well as in angiogenesis through the action of vascular endothelial growth factor.[40] Periostin is elevated in patients with CRSwNP regardless of asthma or atopic comorbidity status and it is especially high in patients with active disease. Conversely, periostin levels seem to decrease after effective treatment and can be helpful in evaluating the efficacy of therapy.[41] Specifically, an established cutoff value of 48.5 ng/mL of s-periostin had a sensitivity of 93.5% for the presence of tissue IL-5. Because periostin seems to regulate protein expression of other inflammatory molecules and tissue remodeling factors, there is potential for periostin itself to serve as a viable target for the reduction of inflammation.[40]

P-glycoprotein

P-glycoprotein is an ATP-dependent transmembrane efflux pump that is upregulated in T_H2 disease, and can cause a portion of CRS-related inflammation through promotion of cytokine secretion.[42,43] It is of particular interest as a biomarker for CRSwNP and as a therapeutic target. P-glycoprotein is also secreted into nasal fluids, making clinical specimen collection and fluid assays more convenient and tolerable for patients than a tissue biopsy. P-glycoprotein levels are elevated in all CRS subtypes, and even higher levels are seen in CRSwNP, specifically with correlation of inferior subjective and objective measures of disease severity with higher levels of P-glycoprotein.[44] Verapamil is an antagonist of p-glycoprotein, and preliminary trials show that low-dose verapamil therapy is safe and effective for CRSwNP treatment. Improvements in SNOT-22 with verapamil resulted in improvements that were comparable with those achieved with steroids or biologic agents.[45]

Immune Cells and Autoantibodies

Immune cell activation and proliferation occurs locally within nasal polyps themselves, with substantially elevated immunoglobulin levels that are not raised at a systemic level. Plasmablasts and plasma cell populations expand rapidly and parallel the growth seen in the T- and B-cell populations in CRSwNP.[46] CXCL-12 and CXCL-13 molecules also are present at increased levels, which enhance B-cell chemotaxis.[47] Type 2 innate lymphoid cells are independently linked with high tissue and blood eosinophilia and are shown to correlate with worse nasal symptom scores.[48] Beyond these cell populations, Tan and colleagues[49] showed IgG and IgA autoantibody elevations within polyp tissue, and the presence of antinuclear, anti-DNA, and anticytokine antibodies is significant. Anti-dsDNA IgG antibody is correlated with a more severe clinical course, whereas the presence of antineutrophil cytoplasmic antibody in patients with CRS may be associated with a subset of individuals difficult-to-treat disease.[50] Autoimmunity and autoantibodies may play a greater role as further work elucidates how these biomarkers may be associated with other phenotypic findings.

Nitric Oxide

It is known that patients with CRSwNP have decrements in exhaled nasal nitric oxide (nNO) owing to ostial occlusion and disruption of gas exchange with the nasal cavity.[51] Patients with CRSsNP also have lower nNO than control patients on average as well, but significantly higher than those observed in CRSwNP.[52] Jeong and colleagues[53] revealed a specific nNO cutoff point with a sensitivity of 81.3% and a specificity of 93.3% for the presence of nasal polyps and, further, nNO levels correlate with the extent of disease.[51,53,54] However, atopic patients in both control groups and patients with nasal polyps have significantly higher nNO levels, confounding some of these findings.[52] Exhaled oral NO is currently used as a marker of asthma control, with lower levels correlating with better disease control. Overall, nNO is a noninvasive biomarker that may have some usefulness for alternative identification of nasal polyp disease and as a marker for disease severity.

Taste Receptors

Over the past several years, a growing body of literature has identified a role for bitter and sweet taste receptors in immune defense in the airway.[55,56] Bitter taste receptors respond to bacterial products, including acyl-homoserine lactones produced by gram-negative bacteria such as *Pseudomonas aeruginosa*.[57] When bitter taste receptors on ciliated cells are stimulated, there is a downstream antimicrobial NO response, resulting in direct bacterial killing and increases in ciliary beat frequency.[58] When a separate cohort of bitter taste receptors on solitary chemosensory cells, another airway cell type, are stimulated, antimicrobial peptides are released.[59] Bitter taste receptors are genetically diverse, and specific genetic polymorphisms correlate with in vitro antimicrobial activity of sinonasal epithelium.[56] This translates to the clinical realm; patients with a nonfunctional polymorphism in a specific taste receptor, T2R38, have inferior outcomes after functional endoscopic sinus surgery and require increased intervention.[60] Furthermore, sinonasal specimens from patients with nonfunctional polymorphisms exhibit increased bacterial biofilm formation.[61] Some in vitro studies also show that bitter taste receptor hyperactivation can be deleterious and potentially proinflammatory, because sinonasal cultures obtained from patients with CRSwNP have increased disease recurrence after sinonasal surgery.

Sweet taste receptors act in opposition to bitter taste receptors, and inhibit the antimicrobial cascade in solitary chemosensory cells. Depletion of airway surface liquid glucose is a harbinger of bacterial infection, because the bacteria consume the sugar rapidly. It is hypothesized that this decrease in glucose deactivates the sweet receptors, which then release their inhibition on the actions of the T2R receptors.[59] Patients with CRS are known to have increased airway glucose levels,[59] similar to those of diabetic patients, who have nasal microbiologic cultures that include far more gram-negative bacteria, including *P aeruginosa*.[62]

Because bitter taste receptors are expressed both on the tongue and in the upper airway, inexpensive phenotypic taste tests can be used as a proxy for the functionality of sinonasal taste receptors. Patients with CRSsNP are significantly more likely to be less sensitive to denatonium, a broad bitter taste receptor agonist, and patients with CRSwNP and CRSsNP are more sensitive to sucrose, which is a sweet receptor agonist.[63] Thus, it may be possible to use bitter and sweet taste tests as biomarkers to evaluate CRS disease status and potentially stratify patients into taste-specific endotypes.

Microbiome

The nasal microbiome is thought to play an important role in the pathogenesis of CRS, and several studies have shown that bacterial diversity is decreased in disease and overall bacterial abundance is increased.[64] This finding suggests that dysbiosis is correlated with CRS status.[65,66] Beyond this, Cope and colleagues[67] demonstrated specific microbiota classifications that correlated with patient phenotypes, including the presence of nasal polyps. A higher than expected proportion of patients with CRSwNP are colonized with *S aureus*,[68] and IgE antibodies to *S aureus* enterotoxins are frequently found in diseased tissue specimens. Both *S aureus* and *P aeruginosa* bacteria can disrupt the epithelial barrier contributing to presumed physiologic mechanisms for CRSwNP development. Compounding the problem, antimicrobial compounds including lysozyme, S100 proteins, and β-defensins all are decreased in patients with CRSwNP compared with matched controls.[69] This reduction in natural defenses could play a key role in shifting the balance toward dysbiosis. Finally, an alternative proposed pathogenic mechanism for T_H2-biased sinusitis is that T cells are allergically sensitized to fungi in the ambient environment, leading to allergic inflammation characterized by a T_H2–high state.[64]

Genetics and Proteomics

Large-scale genetic and proteomic studies hold promise for CRS biomarker identification. It is known that first-degree relatives of patients with CRSwNP have a 4-fold increased risk of developing nasal polyps themselves, but no specific mutation or polymorphism has been individually explanatory, other than those for cystic fibrosis mutations.[70] Genetics are also known to play an important role in other eosinophilic diseases, including eosinophilic esophagitis, suggestive of an inherent predilection to eosinophilia.[71] Gene expression patterns, rather than genetic polymorphisms themselves, are of particular interest. Liu and colleagues[72] revealed 192 upregulated and 156 downregulated genes in polyp tissue using DNA microarray methods. Altered transcription factors include Foxp3 and SOCS3, involved in T-cell regulation,[73] and GATA-3, a T_H2 transcription factor that has been leveraged in early therapeutic trials to decrease asthmatic responses.

Proteomics analysis by Upton and colleagues[74] showed 300 differentially expressed mucosal proteins in patients with CRSwNP compared with matched controls. A separate study identified an even larger cohort of differentially expressed proteins, including mucin 5B, lipocalin-1, mucin 5AC, and arfinase-1. These latter proteins were elevated specifically in patients with nasal polyps.[75] The possibility of proteomic analyses on nasal lavage fluids offers a noninvasive way to obtain a set of secreted biomarkers with potentially rich information.

Other biomarkers

Matrix metalloproteinases are involved in tissue remodeling and are increased specifically in nasal polyp disease. Doxycycline has an anti–matrix metalloproteinase effect that lowers matrix metalloproteinase levels in secretions and causes decreases in polyp size.[76] This property makes doxycycline a potentially beneficial antibiotic choice, whereas other antibiotics such as clarithromycin are more targeted to neutrophilic disease.[77,78] Other compounds of interest include Oncostatin M, an IL-6 related molecule, that is elevated in CRSwNP and causes increased tissue permeability in in vitro sinonasal epithelial cells.[79]

ENDOTYPE CLASSIFICATION

Endotype classification of patients with CRS can use many of these biomarkers to attempt to identify nonphenotypic patient cohorts. This process is not merely an academic exercise; tailored medical and surgical interventions spare an inordinate amount of patient morbidity and unnecessary treatment. If endotype-specific drugs are used, but patients are selected for treatment based only on phenotype, then this patient selection approach may result in many incompletely or inappropriately treated individuals. For example, CRSsNP disease with prominent fibrosis can show severe scarring after aggressive sinonasal surgery, whereas highly eosinophilic CRSwNP disease is much more appropriately treated aggressively. It is thought that aggressive surgery for this extremely eosinophilic endotype of nasal polyp disease eliminates local immune memory and that this intervention is associated with a recurrence-free interval after sinonasal surgery.[80] This is just one example. For the practicing rhinologist, patient subclassification allows for guided preoperative treatment, appropriate surgical management, and improved long-term maintenance.

There are many ways to define patient endotypes. Tomassen and colleagues[17] performed a cluster analysis of patients with CRS with a clinical phenotype-free approach, aiming to identify inflammatory endotypes with immune markers alone. This resulted in 10 defined clusters, generally segregating into 4 clusters with low IL-5 concentrations, eosinophilic cationic protein, and IgE and 6 clusters with increased levels of these compounds. Interestingly, increased IL-5 expression was observed in clusters containing high and low proportions of nasal polyp patients, whereas 1 of the 4 IL-5–negative clusters had a mixed CRSsNP and CRSwNP phenotype with a T_H17 profile. S aureus enterotoxin-specific IgE was observed in all patients with high IL-5 levels and a clinical polyp phenotype. Overall, the study suggests that patient classification by inflammatory endotype provides a more accurate description of the disease than phenotype alone, and that there is a high degree of diversity in CRS inflammation. Although certain inflammatory markers segregate together more frequently, it may be a more multidimensionally heterogeneous disease than previously thought, with separation on T-helper subtype, eosinophilic, and antigenic parameters.

Although not uniformly nonphenotypic, 2 recent studies have identified CRS clusters based on disease characteristics. Soler and colleagues[81] used patient-reported outcome measures after medical and surgical therapy for clustering, identifying a cohort of patients with failure to improve after surgical therapy. A follow-up study proved that these clusters could be applied to a larger, prospective cohort, and that differences in outcomes could be identified in patients treated surgically and those who continued with medical treatment.[82] A second study by Wu and colleagues[83] clustered 110 patients into 3 distinct groups based on course of disease with clinical, functional, and inflammatory parameters. These schema for patient classification may have high usefulness in identifying subsets of patients with a predilection for recalcitrant disease.

SUMMARY

CRS, and specifically CRSwNP, is a substantially heterogeneous disease that exists on a multidimensional spectrum of inflammatory pathology. Endotyping helps to explain some of the differences in clinical manifestations of disease, as well as the variations in therapeutic response and prognosis. Biomarkers provide critical information for endotyping, and it is likely that a panel of CRS biomarkers will be necessary to fully identify T_H2 status associated with nasal polyposis and can be used to guide appropriate therapeutic intervention. The use of high throughput-based studies to identify inflammatory endotypes based on genomics and proteomics holds promise for a future with more accurate CRS diagnosis and tailored medical therapy.

REFERENCES

1. Bachert C, Akdis CA. Phenotypes and emerging endotypes of chronic rhinosinusitis. J Allergy Clin Immunol Pract 2016;4(4):621–8.
2. Stevens WW, Schleimer RP, Kern RC. Chronic rhinosinusitis with nasal polyps. J Allergy Clin Immunol Pract 2016;4(4):565–72.
3. Fokkens WJ, Lund VJ, Mullol J, et al. European position paper on rhinosinusitis and nasal polyps 2012. Rhinol Suppl 2012;23. 3 p preceding table of contents, 1-298.
4. Stevens WW, Ocampo CJ, Berdnikovs S, et al. Cytokines in chronic rhinosinusitis. Role in eosinophilia and aspirin-exacerbated respiratory disease. Am J Respir Crit Care Med 2015;192(6):682–94.
5. Jarvis D, Newson R, Lotvall J, et al. Asthma in adults and its association with chronic rhinosinusitis: the GA2LEN survey in Europe. Allergy 2012;67(1):91–8.
6. Watelet JB, Dogne JM, Mullier F. Remodeling and repair in rhinosinusitis. Curr Allergy Asthma Rep 2015;15(6):34.
7. Soyka MB, Wawrzyniak P, Eiwegger T, et al. Defective epithelial barrier in chronic rhinosinusitis: the regulation of tight junctions by IFN-gamma and IL-4. J Allergy Clin Immunol 2012;130(5):1087–96.e10.
8. Hamilos DL, Leung DY, Muro S, et al. GRbeta expression in nasal polyp inflammatory cells and its relationship to the anti-inflammatory effects of intranasal fluticasone. J Allergy Clin Immunol 2001;108(1):59–68.
9. Wen W, Liu W, Zhang L, et al. Increased neutrophilia in nasal polyps reduces the response to oral corticosteroid therapy. J Allergy Clin Immunol 2012;129(6): 1522–8.e5.
10. Ikeda K, Shiozawa A, Ono N, et al. Subclassification of chronic rhinosinusitis with nasal polyp based on eosinophil and neutrophil. Laryngoscope 2013;123(11): E1–9.
11. Wang X, Zhang N, Bo M, et al. Diversity of TH cytokine profiles in patients with chronic rhinosinusitis: a multicenter study in Europe, Asia, and Oceania. J Allergy Clin Immunol 2016;138(5):1344–53.
12. Ottaviano G, Cappellesso R, Mylonakis I, et al. Endoglin (CD105) expression in sinonasal polyposis. Eur Arch Otorhinolaryngol 2015;272(11):3367–73.
13. Kountakis SE, Arango P, Bradley D, et al. Molecular and cellular staging for the severity of chronic rhinosinusitis. Laryngoscope 2004;114(11):1895–905.

14. Soler ZM, Sauer D, Mace J, et al. Impact of mucosal eosinophilia and nasal polyposis on quality-of-life outcomes after sinus surgery. Otolaryngol Head Neck Surg 2010;142(1):64–71.

15. Steinke JW, Smith AR, Carpenter DJ, et al. Lack of efficacy of symptoms and medical history in distinguishing the degree of eosinophilia in nasal polyps. J Allergy Clin Immunol Pract 2017;5(6):1582–8.e3.

16. Zuo K, Guo J, Chen F, et al. Clinical characteristics and surrogate markers of eosinophilic chronic rhinosinusitis in Southern China. Eur Arch Otorhinolaryngol 2014;271(9):2461–8.

17. Tomassen P, Vandeplas G, Van Zele T, et al. Inflammatory endotypes of chronic rhinosinusitis based on cluster analysis of biomarkers. J Allergy Clin Immunol 2016;137(5):1449–56.e4.

18. Chen JB, James LK, Davies AM, et al. Antibodies and superantibodies in patients with chronic rhinosinusitis with nasal polyps. J Allergy Clin Immunol 2017;139(4):1195–204.e11.

19. Gevaert P, Calus L, Van Bruaene N, et al. Allergic sensitization, high local IL-5 and IgE predict surgical outcome 12 years after endoscopic sinus surgery for chronic rhinosinusitis with nasal polyposis. J Allergy Clin Immunol 2015;135(AB238).

20. Gevaert P, Calus L, Van Zele T, et al. Omalizumab is effective in allergic and nonallergic patients with nasal polyps and asthma. J Allergy Clin Immunol 2013;131(1):110–6.e1.

21. Wise SK, Laury AM, Katz EH, et al. Interleukin-4 and interleukin-13 compromise the sinonasal epithelial barrier and perturb intercellular junction protein expression. Int Forum Allergy Rhinol 2014;4(5):361–70.

22. Kuperman DA, Huang X, Koth LL, et al. Direct effects of interleukin-13 on epithelial cells cause airway hyperreactivity and mucus overproduction in asthma. Nat Med 2002;8(8):885–9.

23. Tan BK, Klingler AI, Poposki JA, et al. Heterogeneous inflammatory patterns in chronic rhinosinusitis without nasal polyps in Chicago, Illinois. J Allergy Clin Immunol 2017;139(2):699–703.e7.

24. Bachert C, Zhang N, Holtappels G, et al. Presence of IL-5 protein and IgE antibodies to staphylococcal enterotoxins in nasal polyps is associated with comorbid asthma. J Allergy Clin Immunol 2010;126(5):962–8, 968.e1–6.

25. Lam M, Hull L, Imrie A, et al. Interleukin-25 and interleukin-33 as mediators of eosinophilic inflammation in chronic rhinosinusitis. Am J Rhinol Allergy 2015;29(3):175–81.

26. Lam M, Hull L, McLachlan R, et al. Clinical severity and epithelial endotypes in chronic rhinosinusitis. Int Forum Allergy Rhinol 2013;3(2):121–8.

27. Chen F, Hong H, Sun Y, et al. Nasal interleukin 25 as a novel biomarker for patients with chronic rhinosinusitis with nasal polyps and airway hypersensitiveness: a pilot study. Ann Allergy Asthma Immunol 2017;119(4):310–6.e2.

28. Ozturan A, Eyigor H, Eyigor M, et al. The role of IL-25 and IL-33 in chronic rhinosinusitis with or without nasal polyps. Eur Arch Otorhinolaryngol 2017;274(1):283–8.

29. FitzGerald JM, Bleecker ER, Nair P, et al. Benralizumab, an anti-interleukin-5 receptor alpha monoclonal antibody, as add-on treatment for patients with severe, uncontrolled, eosinophilic asthma (CALIMA): a randomised, double-blind, placebo-controlled phase 3 trial. Lancet 2016;388(10056):2128–41.

30. Gevaert P, Van Bruaene N, Cattaert T, et al. Mepolizumab, a humanized anti-IL-5 mAb, as a treatment option for severe nasal polyposis. J Allergy Clin Immunol 2011;128(5):989–95.e1–8.

31. Bachert C, Sousa AR, Lund VJ, et al. Reduced need for surgery in severe nasal polyposis with mepolizumab: randomized trial. J Allergy Clin Immunol 2017; 140(4):1024–31.e14.

32. Naclerio RM, Baroody FM, Pinto JM. Nasal polyps and biomarkers. J Allergy Clin Immunol Pract 2017;5(6):1589–90.

33. Wenzel S, Castro M, Corren J, et al. Dupilumab efficacy and safety in adults with uncontrolled persistent asthma despite use of medium-to-high-dose inhaled corticosteroids plus a long-acting beta2 agonist: a randomised double-blind placebo-controlled pivotal phase 2b dose-ranging trial. Lancet 2016;388(10039): 31–44.

34. Bachert C, Mannent L, Naclerio RM, et al. Effect of subcutaneous dupilumab on nasal polyp burden in patients with chronic sinusitis and nasal polyposis: a randomized clinical trial. JAMA 2016;315(5):469–79.

35. Hanania NA, Noonan M, Corren J, et al. Lebrikizumab in moderate-to-severe asthma: pooled data from two randomised placebo-controlled studies. Thorax 2015;70(8):748–56.

36. Shin HW, Kim DK, Park MH, et al. IL-25 as a novel therapeutic target in nasal polyps of patients with chronic rhinosinusitis. J Allergy Clin Immunol 2015; 135(6):1476–85.e7.

37. Oyer SL, Mulligan JK, Psaltis AJ, et al. Cytokine correlation between sinus tissue and nasal secretions among chronic rhinosinusitis and controls. Laryngoscope 2013;123(12):E72–8.

38. Dupilumab (Dupixent) for moderate to severe atopic dermatitis. Med Lett Drugs Ther 2017;59(1519):64–6.

39. Wang M, Wang X, Zhang N, et al. Association of periostin expression with eosinophilic inflammation in nasal polyps. J Allergy Clin Immunol 2015;136(6): 1700–3.e9.

40. Xu M, Chen D, Zhou H, et al. The role of periostin in the occurrence and progression of eosinophilic chronic sinusitis with nasal polyps. Sci Rep 2017;7(1):9479.

41. Kim DW, Kulka M, Jo A, et al. Cross-talk between human mast cells and epithelial cells by IgE-mediated periostin production in eosinophilic nasal polyps. J Allergy Clin Immunol 2017;139(5):1692–5.e6.

42. Bleier BS. Regional expression of epithelial MDR1/P-glycoprotein in chronic rhinosinusitis with and without nasal polyposis. Int Forum Allergy Rhinol 2012;2(2): 122–5.

43. Feldman RE, Lam AC, Sadow PM, et al. P-glycoprotein is a marker of tissue eosinophilia and radiographic inflammation in chronic rhinosinusitis without nasal polyps. Int Forum Allergy Rhinol 2013;3(8):684–7.

44. Nocera AL, Meurer AT, Miyake MM, et al. Secreted P-glycoprotein is a noninvasive biomarker of chronic rhinosinusitis. Laryngoscope 2017;127(1):E1–4.

45. Miyake MM, Nocera A, Levesque P, et al. Double-blind placebo-controlled randomized clinical trial of verapamil for chronic rhinosinusitis with nasal polyps. J Allergy Clin Immunol 2017;140(1):271–3.

46. Hulse KE, Norton JE, Suh L, et al. Chronic rhinosinusitis with nasal polyps is characterized by B-cell inflammation and EBV-induced protein 2 expression. J Allergy Clin Immunol 2013;131(4):1075–83, 1083.e1–7.

47. Peters AT, Kato A, Zhang N, et al. Evidence for altered activity of the IL-6 pathway in chronic rhinosinusitis with nasal polyps. J Allergy Clin Immunol 2010;125(2): 397–403.e10.

48. Ho J, Bailey M, Zaunders J, et al. Group 2 innate lymphoid cells (ILC2s) are increased in chronic rhinosinusitis with nasal polyps or eosinophilia. Clin Exp Allergy 2015;45(2):394–403.
49. Tan BK, Li QZ, Suh L, et al. Evidence for intranasal antinuclear autoantibodies in patients with chronic rhinosinusitis with nasal polyps. J Allergy Clin Immunol 2011;128(6):1198–206.e1.
50. Goncalves C, Pinaffi JV, Carvalho JF, et al. Antineutrophil cytoplasmic antibodies in chronic rhinosinusitis may be a marker of undisclosed vasculitis. Am J Rhinol 2007;21(6):691–4.
51. Delclaux C, Malinvaud D, Chevalier-Bidaud B, et al. Nitric oxide evaluation in upper and lower respiratory tracts in nasal polyposis. Clin Exp Allergy 2008;38(7):1140–7.
52. Liu C, Zheng M, He F, et al. Role of exhaled nasal nitric oxide in distinguishing between chronic rhinosinusitis with and without nasal polyps. Am J Rhinol Allergy 2017;31(6):389–94.
53. Jeong JH, Yoo HS, Lee SH, et al. Nasal and exhaled nitric oxide in chronic rhinosinusitis with polyps. Am J Rhinol Allergy 2014;28(1):e11–6.
54. Lee JM, McKnight CL, Aves T, et al. Nasal nitric oxide as a marker of sinus mucosal health in patients with nasal polyposis. Int Forum Allergy Rhinol 2015;5(10):894–9.
55. Tizzano M, Gulbransen BD, Vandenbeuch A, et al. Nasal chemosensory cells use bitter taste signaling to detect irritants and bacterial signals. Proc Natl Acad Sci U S A 2010;107(7):3210–5.
56. Lee RJ, Xiong G, Kofonow JM, et al. T2R38 taste receptor polymorphisms underlie susceptibility to upper respiratory infection. J Clin Invest 2012;122(11):4145–59.
57. Jimenez PN, Koch G, Thompson JA, et al. The multiple signaling systems regulating virulence in Pseudomonas aeruginosa. Microbiol Mol Biol Rev 2012;76(1):46–65.
58. Shah AS, Ben-Shahar Y, Moninger TO, et al. Motile cilia of human airway epithelia are chemosensory. Science 2009;325(5944):1131–4.
59. Lee RJ, Kofonow JM, Rosen PL, et al. Bitter and sweet taste receptors regulate human upper respiratory innate immunity. J Clin Invest 2014;124(3):1393–405.
60. Adappa ND, Zhang Z, Palmer JN, et al. The bitter taste receptor T2R38 is an independent risk factor for chronic rhinosinusitis requiring sinus surgery. Int Forum Allergy Rhinol 2014;4(1):3–7.
61. Adappa ND, Truesdale CM, Workman AD, et al. Correlation of T2R38 taste phenotype and in vitro biofilm formation from nonpolypoid chronic rhinosinusitis patients. Int Forum Allergy Rhinol 2016;6(8):783–91.
62. Zhang Z, Adappa ND, Lautenbach E, et al. The effect of diabetes mellitus on chronic rhinosinusitis and sinus surgery outcome. Int Forum Allergy Rhinol 2014;4(4):315–20.
63. Workman AD, Brooks SG, Kohanski MA, et al. Bitter and sweet taste tests are reflective of disease status in chronic rhinosinusitis. J Allergy Clin Immunol Pract 2018. https://doi.org/10.1016/j.jaip.2017.09.014.
64. Mahdavinia M, Keshavarzian A, Tobin MC, et al. A comprehensive review of the nasal microbiome in chronic rhinosinusitis (CRS). Clin Exp Allergy 2016;46(1):21–41.
65. Boase S, Foreman A, Cleland E, et al. The microbiome of chronic rhinosinusitis: culture, molecular diagnostics and biofilm detection. BMC Infect Dis 2013;13:210.

66. Hoggard M, Biswas K, Zoing M, et al. Evidence of microbiota dysbiosis in chronic rhinosinusitis. Int Forum Allergy Rhinol 2017;7(3):230–9.
67. Cope EK, Goldberg AN, Pletcher SD, et al. Compositionally and functionally distinct sinus microbiota in chronic rhinosinusitis patients have immunological and clinically divergent consequences. Microbiome 2017;5(1):53.
68. Malik Z, Roscioli E, Murphy J, et al. Staphylococcus aureus impairs the airway epithelial barrier in vitro. Int Forum Allergy Rhinol 2015;5(6):551–6.
69. Seshadri S, Lin DC, Rosati M, et al. Reduced expression of antimicrobial PLUNC proteins in nasal polyp tissues of patients with chronic rhinosinusitis. Allergy 2012;67(7):920–8.
70. Oakley GM, Curtin K, Orb Q, et al. Familial risk of chronic rhinosinusitis with and without nasal polyposis: genetics or environment. Int Forum Allergy Rhinol 2015; 5(4):276–82.
71. Schleimer RP. Immunopathogenesis of chronic rhinosinusitis and nasal polyposis. Annu Rev Pathol 2017;12:331–57.
72. Liu Z, Kim J, Sypek JP, et al. Gene expression profiles in human nasal polyp tissues studied by means of DNA microarray. J Allergy Clin Immunol 2004;114(4): 783–90.
73. Lan F, Zhang N, Zhang J, et al. Forkhead box protein 3 in human nasal polyp regulatory T cells is regulated by the protein suppressor of cytokine signaling 3. J Allergy Clin Immunol 2013;132(6):1314–21.
74. Upton DC, Welham NV, Kuo JS, et al. Chronic rhinosinusitis with nasal polyps: a proteomic analysis. Annals of Otology, Rhinology & Laryngology 2011;120(12): 780–6.
75. Lee M, Kim DW, Kim YM, et al. In-depth High-resolution Proteomic Analysis Using Nasal Secretions form Chronic Rhinosinusitis and Nasal Polyps. J Allergy Clin Immunol 2017;139(2):AB179.
76. Pinto Bezerra Soter AC, Bezerra TF, Pezato R, et al. Prospective open-label evaluation of long-term low-dose doxycycline for difficult-to-treat chronic rhinosinusitis with nasal polyps. Rhinology 2017;55(2):175–80.
77. Fokkens WJ, Lund VJ, Mullol J, et al. EPOS 2012: European position paper on rhinosinusitis and nasal polyps 2012. A summary for otorhinolaryngologists. Rhinology 2012;50(1):1–12.
78. Van Zele T, Gevaert P, Holtappels G, et al. Oral steroids and doxycycline: two different approaches to treat nasal polyps. J Allergy Clin Immunol 2010;125(5): 1069–76.e4.
79. Pothoven KL, Norton JE, Hulse KE, et al. Oncostatin M promotes mucosal epithelial barrier dysfunction, and its expression is increased in patients with eosinophilic mucosal disease. J Allergy Clin Immunol 2015;136(3):737–46.e4.
80. Bassiouni A, Wormald PJ. Role of frontal sinus surgery in nasal polyp recurrence. Laryngoscope 2013;123(1):36–41.
81. Soler ZM, Hyer JM, Ramakrishnan V, et al. Identification of chronic rhinosinusitis phenotypes using cluster analysis. Int Forum Allergy Rhinol 2015;5(5):399–407.
82. Soler ZM, Hyer JM, Rudmik L, et al. Cluster analysis and prediction of treatment outcomes for chronic rhinosinusitis. J Allergy Clin Immunol 2016;137(4):1054–62.
83. Wu D, Bleier BS, Li L, et al. Clinical phenotypes of nasal polyps and comorbid asthma based on cluster analysis of disease history. J Allergy Clin Immunol Pract 2017. https://doi.org/10.1016/j.jaip.2017.09.020.

UNITED STATES POSTAL SERVICE ® — Statement of Ownership, Management, and Circulation (All Periodicals Publications Except Requester Publications)

1. Publication Title
IMMUNOLOGY AND ALLERGY CLINICS OF NORTH AMERICA

2. Publication Number
006 – 361

3. Filing Date
9/18/2018

4. Issue Frequency
FEB, MAY, AUG, NOV

5. Number of Issues Published Annually
4

6. Annual Subscription Price
$333.00

7. Complete Mailing Address of Known Office of Publication (Not printer) (Street, city, county, state, and ZIP+4®)
ELSEVIER INC.
230 Park Avenue, Suite 800
New York, NY 10169

Contact Person
STEPHEN R. BUSHING
Telephone (Include area code)
215-239-3688

8. Complete Mailing Address of Headquarters or General Business Office of Publisher (Not printer)
ELSEVIER INC.
230 Park Avenue, Suite 800
New York, NY 10169

9. Full Names and Complete Mailing Addresses of Publisher, Editor, and Managing Editor (Do not leave blank)

Publisher (Name and complete mailing address)
TAYLOR E. BALL, ELSEVIER INC.
1600 JOHN F KENNEDY BLVD. SUITE 1800
PHILADELPHIA, PA 19103-2899

Editor (Name and complete mailing address)
JESSICA MCCOOL, ELSEVIER INC.
1600 JOHN F KENNEDY BLVD. SUITE 1800
PHILADELPHIA, PA 19103-2899

Managing Editor (Name and complete mailing address)
PATRICK MANLEY, ELSEVIER INC.
1600 JOHN F KENNEDY BLVD. SUITE 1800
PHILADELPHIA, PA 19103-2899

10. Owner (Do not leave blank. If the publication is owned by a corporation, give the name and address of the corporation immediately followed by the names and addresses of all stockholders owning or holding 1 percent or more of the total amount of stock. If not owned by a corporation, give the names and addresses of the individual owners. If owned by a partnership or other unincorporated firm, give its name and address as well as those of each individual owner. If the publication is published by a nonprofit organization, give its name and address.)

Full Name	Complete Mailing Address
WHOLLY OWNED SUBSIDIARY OF REED/ELSEVIER, US HOLDINGS	1600 JOHN F KENNEDY BLVD. SUITE 1800 PHILADELPHIA, PA 19103-2899

11. Known Bondholders, Mortgagees, and Other Security Holders Owning or Holding 1 Percent or More of Total Amount of Bonds, Mortgages, or Other Securities. If none, check box. ▶ ☐ None

Full Name	Complete Mailing Address
N/A	

12. Tax Status (For completion by nonprofit organizations authorized to mail at nonprofit rates) (Check one)
The purpose, function, and nonprofit status of this organization and the exempt status for federal income tax purposes:
☒ Has Not Changed During Preceding 12 Months
☐ Has Changed During Preceding 12 Months (Publisher must submit explanation of change with this statement)

PS Form **3526**, July 2014 [Page 1 of 4 (see instructions page 4)] PSN: 7530-01-000-9931 PRIVACY NOTICE: See our privacy policy on www.usps.com

---

13. Publication Title
IMMUNOLOGY AND ALLERGY CLINICS OF NORTH AMERICA

14. Issue Date for Circulation Data Below
MAY 2018

15. Extent and Nature of Circulation			Average No. Copies Each Issue During Preceding 12 Months	No. Copies of Single Issue Published Nearest to Filing Date
a. Total Number of Copies (Net press run)			133	213
b. Paid Circulation (By Mail and Outside the Mail)	(1)	Mailed Outside-County Paid Subscriptions Stated on PS Form 3541 (Include paid distribution above nominal rate, advertiser's proof copies, and exchange copies)	74	107
	(2)	Mailed In-County Paid Subscriptions Stated on PS Form 3541 (Include paid distribution above nominal rate, advertiser's proof copies, and exchange copies)	0	0
	(3)	Paid Distribution Outside the Mails Including Sales Through Dealers and Carriers, Street Vendors, Counter Sales, and Other Paid Distribution Outside USPS®	20	29
	(4)	Paid Distribution by Other Classes of Mail Through the USPS (e.g. First-Class Mail®)	0	0
c. Total Paid Distribution [Sum of 15b (1), (2), (3), and (4)]			94	136
d. Free or Nominal Rate Distribution (By Mail and Outside the Mail)	(1)	Free or Nominal Rate Outside-County Copies included on PS Form 3541	29	61
	(2)	Free or Nominal Rate In-County Copies Included on PS Form 3541	0	0
	(3)	Free or Nominal Rate Copies Mailed at Other Classes Through the USPS (e.g., First-Class Mail)	0	0
	(4)	Free or Nominal Rate Distribution Outside the Mail (Carriers or other means)	29	61
e. Total Free or Nominal Rate Distribution (Sum of 15d (1), (2), (3) and (4))			29	61
f. Total Distribution (Sum of 15c and 15e)			123	197
g. Copies not Distributed (See Instructions to Publishers #4 (page 83))			10	16
h. Total (Sum of 15f and g)			133	213
i. Percent Paid (15c divided by 15f times 100)			76.42%	69.04%

* If you are claiming electronic copies, go to line 16 on page 3. If you are not claiming electronic copies, skip to line 17 on page 3.

16. Electronic Copy Circulation	Average No. Copies Each Issue During Preceding 12 Months	No. Copies of Single Issue Published Nearest to Filing Date
a. Paid Electronic Copies ▶	0	0
b. Total Paid Print Copies (Line 15c) + Paid Electronic Copies (Line 16a) ▶	94	136
c. Total Print Distribution (Line 15f) + Paid Electronic Copies (Line 16a) ▶	123	197
d. Percent Paid (Both Print & Electronic Copies) (16b divided by 16c × 100) ▶	76.42%	69.04%

☒ I certify that 60% of all my distributed copies (electronic and print) are paid above a nominal price.

17. Publication of Statement of Ownership
☒ If the publication is a general publication, publication of this statement is required. Will be printed
in the NOVEMBER 2018 issue of this publication.
☐ Publication not required.

18. Signature and Title of Editor, Publisher, Business Manager, or Owner
STEPHEN R. BUSHING - INVENTORY DISTRIBUTION CONTROL MANAGER

[signature] Stephen R. Bushing Date 9/18/2018

I certify that all information furnished on this form is true and complete. I understand that anyone who furnishes false or misleading information on this form or who omits material or information requested on the form may be subject to criminal sanctions (including fines and imprisonment) and/or civil sanctions (including civil penalties).

PS Form **3526**, July 2014 (Page 3 of 4) PRIVACY NOTICE: See our privacy policy on www.usps.com

Moving?

Make sure your subscription moves with you!

To notify us of your new address, find your **Clinics Account Number** (located on your mailing label above your name), and contact customer service at:

Email: journalscustomerservice-usa@elsevier.com

800-654-2452 (subscribers in the U.S. & Canada)
314-447-8871 (subscribers outside of the U.S. & Canada)

Fax number: 314-447-8029

Elsevier Health Sciences Division
Subscription Customer Service
3251 Riverport Lane
Maryland Heights, MO 63043

*To ensure uninterrupted delivery of your subscription, please notify us at least 4 weeks in advance of move.

Printed and bound by CPI Group (UK) Ltd, Croydon, CR0 4YY

03/10/2024

01040397-0013